CHILDREN AND
ENVIRONMENTAL TOXINS

WHAT EVERYONE NEEDS TO KNOW®

CHILDREN AND ENVIRONMENTAL TOXINS

WHAT EVERYONE NEEDS TO KNOW®

PHILIP J. LANDRIGAN, MD, MSC, FAAP
MARY M. LANDRIGAN, MPA

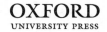

OXFORD
UNIVERSITY PRESS

OXFORD
UNIVERSITY PRESS

Oxford University Press is a department of the University of Oxford. It furthers
the University's objective of excellence in research, scholarship, and education
by publishing worldwide. Oxford is a registered trade mark of Oxford University
Press in the UK and certain other countries.

"What Everyone Needs to Know" is a registered trademark
of Oxford University Press.

You must not circulate this work in any other form
and you must impose this same condition on any acquirer.

Published in the United States of America by Oxford University Press
198 Madison Avenue, New York, NY 10016, United States of America.

© Oxford University Press 2018

Library of Congress Cataloging-in-Publication Data
Names: Landrigan, Philip J., author. | Landrigan, Mary M.
Title: Children and environmental toxins : what everyone needs to know /
Philip J. Landrigan, Mary M. Landrigan.
Description: Oxford ; New York : Oxford University Press, 2018. |
Series: What everyone needs to know |
Includes bibliographical references and index.
Identifiers: LCCN 2017025622 | ISBN 9780190662639 (paperback) |
ISBN 9780190662646 (hardcover)
Subjects: LCSH: Environmentally induced diseases in children—United States. |
Pediatric toxicology—United States. | Children—
Health and hygiene—United States. | BISAC: HEALTH & FITNESS /
General. | MEDICAL / Public Health.
Classification: LCC RA1225 .L35 2017 | DDC 616.9/80083—dc23
LC record available at https://lccn.loc.gov/2017025622

1 3 5 7 9 8 6 4 2

Paperback printed by LSC Communications, United States of America
Hardback printed by Bridgeport National Bindery, Inc., United States of America

To our children,
Mary and Jacob; Chris and Clare; and Lizzie and Raphael;

To their children,
Jack, Ryan, Mary Katya, Sara, Gabriel, Aelish, and Isaac;

And to their children's children

CONTENTS

3. Children's Unique Vulnerability to Toxic Chemicals in the Environment   25

4. The Links Between Toxic Chemicals in the Environment and Disease in Children   35

5. Lead in the Home   73

10. Toxic Chemicals and Other Hazards in the Home   143

11. Daycare   155

ABOUT THE AUTHORS

Philip J. Landrigan, MD, MSc, is a pediatrician, epidemiologist, and internationally recognized pioneer in children's environmental health. His studies of childhood lead poisoning catalyzed the removal lead from gasoline—an action that reduced childhood lead poisoning in the United States by over 90% and has raised the IQ of children around the world. His studies on children's vulnerability to pesticides triggered passage of the Food Quality Protection Act, the federal pesticide law, the only US environmental law with standards explicitly protecting the health of children. He has been a leader in the US National Children's Study. He has consulted to the World Health Organization, published seven books, and written over 600 scientific articles.

Mary M. Landrigan, MPA, is a nationally known public health educator and former health care administrator with 25 years of experience at the Westchester County Department of Health. Her special expertise is translating current scientific and medical research into health messages for parents and community members. She is co-author of *Raising Healthy Children in a Toxic World* (Rodale Press, 2002) together with Dr. Philip Landrigan and Dr. Herbert Needleman. She has been active in local environmental advocacy and legislative issues in New York State and is a former president of the New York Public Health Association.

INTRODUCTION

Children today live longer, healthier lives and suffer less disease than children at any previous time in history. A child born this year in the United States, Canada, Great Britain, Germany, France, Australia, Italy, or Japan can expect to live for 80 years and more—nearly double the 45- to 50-year life span that was the norm only 100 years ago at the beginning of the 20th century.

This unprecedented gain in health and longevity is a triumph for modern medicine and public health. It reflects the success of vaccines and antibiotics, the widespread availability of healthy food and safe drinking water, a 90% reduction in infant mortality, and control of the ancient infectious diseases—cholera, smallpox, typhus, yellow fever, scarlet fever, tuberculosis, measles, malaria, pertussis, and polio—that previously decimated the world's children. It is a great step forward for humanity.

But two negative developments overshadow this extraordinary progress and threaten to undo it.

First is the invention and wide dissemination into the modern environment of tens of thousands of new chemicals—new materials that never before existed in nature nor were found in the earth's environment. These man-made, synthetic chemicals are used today in millions of consumer products. They have migrated to the most remote corners of the planet. Some are highly persistent and will remain in soil and water for decades, if not centuries. These chemicals get into people, including infants and children. Surveys conducted in the United States by the Centers for Disease Control and Prevention (CDC) routinely detect more than 200 synthetic chemicals in the bodies of nearly all Americans, even in the breast milk of nursing mothers and in the umbilical cord blood of newborn infants.

The second negative development is the rise of noncommunicable disease. Over the past 50 years, noncommunicable diseases and disorders have become epidemic among the world's children. They have replaced the infectious diseases as major causes of disability and death. And they are on the rise. Here are some key statistics:

- Childhood asthma has nearly tripled in frequency since the early 1970s.
- Learning disabilities affect 1 child in 6. One of every 68 children born in America is now diagnosed with autism spectrum disorder, according to the CDC.
- Leukemia and brain cancer, the two main types of pediatric cancer, have both increased in incidence by nearly 40% since the early 1970s. Despite tremendous advances in cancer treatment, cancer is now the leading cause of disease death among children.
- Certain birth defects have doubled in frequency, and birth defects have become the leading cause of death in infancy.
- Childhood obesity has more than tripled since the 1970s—today nearly 1 child in 5 in America is obese.
- Type 2 diabetes, previously an adult disease, has become epidemic among children and is diagnosed at ever earlier ages.

The epidemic of noncommunicable disease in children began in North America, Western Europe, and other highly developed countries, but it is now spreading worldwide. Rising rates of asthma, cancer, birth defects, and obesity are seen today among children in India and China and also in parts of Latin America and Africa that only a generation ago knew starvation and famine. The global pandemic of noncommunicable disease in the world's children is one of the great health problems of our time. If it is not checked, it threatens to undo all of the great gains that medicine and public health have made in the past century.

Toxic chemicals are important causes of noncommunicable disease in children. Toxic chemicals in air, water, soil, household products, and breast milk expose children to health threats that can cause lifelong damage. Research in children's environmental health and epidemiology shows us that infants and children are exquisitely vulnerable to toxic chemicals. Exposures during pregnancy and in early childhood to even very low levels of lead, methylmercury, organophosphate pesticides, and polychlorinated biphenyls (PCBs) have all been proven to cause damage to children's developing brains that presents as IQ loss, shortened attention span, and disordered behavior. Early-life exposure to air pollution causes asthma, pneumonia, impaired lung growth, and sudden infant death. Prenatal exposures to solvents and pesticides are linked to childhood cancer. Endocrine disruptors, such as phthalates and bisphenol A, are associated with birth defects, diminished reproductive function, and disordered behavior. Toxic chemical exposures cause disease in children at exposure levels far lower than in adults.

Despite great recent gains in knowledge of the effects of toxic chemicals on children's health, there is an enormous amount we still do not know. For example, many of the chemicals in widest use today have never been tested for safety or toxicity. Fewer still have been assessed for their potential to disrupt early human development. Without safety testing data, there is no way to know whether a chemical may injure children or how it may do so.

Although many of us rely on governmental regulations to protect us from the harms of chemicals, the reality is that in many countries the protections are inadequate and do not protect children against dangers of toxic chemicals. Most governments around the world, including the United States, have simply presumed that new chemicals are safe until they are conclusively proven to cause harm, and these countries have required little or no premarket testing of most chemicals. Only a few governments, notably the European Union, through its 2007 REACH legislation, have attempted to establish chemical safety legislation designed to protect children's health and the environment.

After many years of debate, the United States passed chemical safety legislation in 2016—the Senator Frank R. Lautenberg Chemical Safety for the 21st Century Act. As of this writing, the new law is only beginning to be implemented—time will tell whether it will protect our children or be diluted and made ineffective, as were earlier efforts to control toxic chemicals in the United States.

In rapidly developing low- and middle-income countries where chemical pollution has become rampant, controls are even weaker, and children's exposures are severe. Consider, for example, urban air pollution in Beijing and New Delhi and arsenic contamination of drinking water in Bangladesh.

As a consequence of the weak chemical control policies that exist today in most countries, people around the world and especially children are exposed on a daily basis to scores of chemicals of unknown hazard. The extent to which toxic chemicals in the environment are contributing to rising rates of autism, childhood cancer, birth defects, learning disabilities and decreased fertility is only beginning to be discerned. And perhaps even more disturbing, we are beginning only now, more than a century after the rise the chemical manufacturing industry, to realize that exposures to toxic chemicals in early life may cause disease and disability not only in childhood, but across the entire life span. Early-life exposures to toxic chemicals are now beginning to be linked to adult-onset hypertension, heart disease, stroke, and cancer, as well as to neurodegenerative diseases, such as Parkinson disease and dementia.

The topics covered in this book span a wide range. The first four chapters offer a crash course for professionals and parents who want to understand how children's bodies are particularly sensitive to their chemical environment. The rest of the book is an individual's guide to understanding chemical toxins in one's own environment: what you can do at home to minimize threats from toxic chemicals in household products; what actions you can take to protect your own reproductive health before and during pregnancy; how you can make your baby's room safe; tips about avoiding allergy and asthma attacks; and cautions about pesticides. You will learn how to choose safer foods and household cleaning agents. These details can be applied to both the home and to places like schools and daycare facilities, and will help to minimize toxic exposures for both children and adults while more permanent societal protections are pursued.

1

THE CHANGING PATTERNS OF DISEASE IN CHILDREN

How have patterns of disease in children changed over the past century?

In 1900, a baby born in the United States could be expected to live to about 45 to 50 years of age. One in three children died before his or her first birthday. Almost all of childhood deaths were due to infectious diseases: now-preventable illnesses like pneumonia, dysentery, cholera, smallpox, typhoid fever, pertussis, and measles.

Figure 1-1 shows that the death rate (the number of deaths per 1,000 people per year) in New York City in 1800 was twice as high as it is today. The reason? Because, on average, in 1800 people could expect to live only about half as long as they live today. To be sure, some people back then lived to a ripe old age, but many babies died in infancy, children died during childhood, and young mothers died in giving birth. Thus the average life span was relatively short.

Life expectancy began to increase during the late 19th and early 20th centuries. The great cities saw dramatic changes in their environments that brought about enormous improvements in health. Engineers constructed reservoirs and aqueducts to bring clean water to the cities, with projects such as the Croton Aqueduct in New York City and the Quabbin Reservoir serving Boston. Sewage systems were constructed

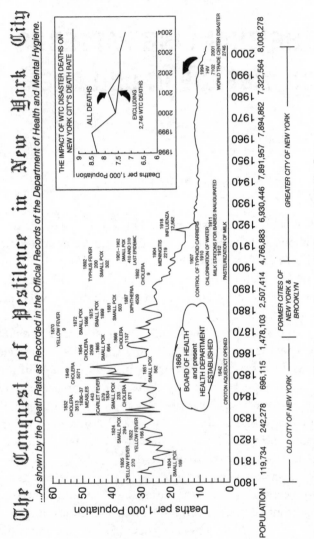

Figure 1-1 Patterns of Disease Change with Development—Environmental Change is the Driving Force

to remove waste. City governments worked to ensure that their people had wholesome food and decent housing. Insects and vermin that spread disease began to be controlled. These environmental changes contributed to the control of cholera, typhoid fever, yellow fever, tuberculosis, and the other ancient infectious diseases. As the graph in Figure 1-1 shows, the death rate began to go steadily down beginning in the 1870s. Overall health improved in spite of the fact that penicillin was not discovered for another 60 years in 1928.

Factors that have continued to drive down rates of disease and death among children in more recent decades include vaccines and antibiotics, improved nutrition, the prevention of premature birth and low birth weight, and all of the high-tech improvements in the care of sick children that are the consequence of advances in modern medicine.

Today, the ancient scourges of tuberculosis, measles, whooping cough, and polio no longer decimate our children in the United States. Life expectancy has risen to nearly 80 years. Infant deaths have fallen by 90% since 1900. Similar health trends have been observed in country after country as nations have moved through the stages of development toward cleaner air, cleaner water, safer food, and control of infectious diseases. Improvements continue into the present. It is unquestionable that the environment has enormous power to shape health and disease in children as well as in adults.

What are the predominant diseases of children today?

Today the major causes of illness of children in the United States, Canada, Japan, Australia, and Western Europe are no longer infectious diseases. Despite the ever-present threats of tuberculosis, AIDS, and emerging infections, such as Ebola and Zika virus infection, the principal causes of disease, disability, and death among children in the industrially developed countries of the world today are noncommunicable diseases— asthma, obesity, learning disabilities, autism, attention deficit/

hyperactivity disorder, and diabetes. All of these diseases and disorders are on the rise:

- **Asthma** prevalence among children in the United States has nearly tripled, from 3.6% in 1980 to almost 10% today. Asthma has become the leading cause of pediatric hospitalization and school absenteeism. In 2010, 9.4% of US children (6.7 million children) were diagnosed with asthma.
- **Birth defects** are now the leading cause of infant death. Certain birth defects, such as hypospadias (malformation of genitals in boys) and gastroschisis (abdominal wall defect where intestines protrude outside the body), are reported by the Centers for Disease Control (CDC) to have increased substantially.
- **Autism spectrum disorder** now affects 1 of every 68 American children. Attention deficit/hyperactivity disorder (ADHD) is diagnosed in 14% of American children, two thirds of whom also have a learning disability. Developmental disorders of the brain, including dyslexia, mental retardation, ADHD, and autism spectrum disorders, affect 400,000 to 600,000 of the 4 million babies born each year in the United States.
- **Leukemia** and **brain cancer** are on the increase. Between the 1970s and the 1990s, the rate of new cases of cancer in children increased by 40%. Although new treatments have lowered the death rate, cancer is now the second leading cause of death in American children, surpassed only by injuries.
- **Testicular cancer** in young men, ages 15 to 30 years, a disease that probably has its origins during fetal life, has more than doubled in incidence and is occurring at younger ages.
- **Type 2 diabetes**, known formerly as adult-onset diabetes, was almost never previously seen in childhood. Now, as childhood obesity increases, type 2 diabetes is

diagnosed among children with increasing frequency and at younger ages.

Evidence is strong and growing that exposures in the environment are important causes of these health problems in children. To understand that evidence, it's important to recognize the changes in the chemical landscape that have coincided with the changes in disease incidence.

2

THE CHEMICAL ENVIRONMENT

What are the origins of the chemical manufacturing industry?

The chemical manufacturing industry had its origins in Germany and Switzerland in the late 19th and early 20th centuries. In the first decades of the 20th century, the industry spread to England, and then in the years before World War II it expanded to North America, Australia, and Japan. Since the 1950s, the industry has spread globally.

Beginning early in the 20th century, toxic chemicals began for the first time to move in substantial quantities from industrial facilities out into the general environment. This was a direct result of the rise and global spread of the chemical manufacturing industry and the introduction of new and untested chemicals into consumer products. Widespread contamination of air, water, and soil with toxic chemicals also began to be seen at that time.

The rapid growth of industrial chemical manufacture has resulted in a wealth of new consumer products and technological advances, many of which have improved our lives and made us safer. But unfortunately, in the haste of production, new, untested, and potentially dangerous chemicals have been incorporated into thousands of household items. Furthermore, older toxins, such as lead and asbestos that were placed in consumer products many years ago continue to be responsible for hazardous exposures in homes and communities. The result has been growth of environmentally caused diseases, including lead poisoning and chemically induced cancers.

When were environmentally caused diseases first observed?

Environmentally caused diseases were first spotted in industrial workers, who because of their work were the first to experience heavy exposure to chemicals in the workplace. Disease in chemical workers has followed the chemical manufacturing industry almost from its beginnings.

Occupational lead poisoning is perhaps the oldest known occupational disease. It was first reported in Roman times among lead miners by Pliny the Elder and by the Greek poet-physician Nikander. Occupational lead poisoning was described in the Middle Ages among lead miners and smelter workers by the German physician Agricola. The clinical symptoms of lead poisoning were described in great detail in the early 1700s by Bernardino Ramazzini, an Italian physician, considered today to be the "father of occupational medicine."

One of the earliest reports of occupational disease caused by synthetic chemicals was an 1898 report of an outbreak of bladder cancer among chemical workers in Switzerland who were occupationally exposed to synthetic aniline dyes, one of the first classes of man-made chemicals. As the chemical and dye manufacturing industry spread globally, bladder cancer followed—first to England and North America and then more broadly. The disease typically made its appearance in a country about 20 years after the start of dye manufacture. Synthetic aniline dyes have now been confirmed to be the cause of bladder cancer, and these chemicals are classified today as proven human carcinogens by the International Agency for Research on Cancer (IARC), the cancer agency of the World Health Organization. The dyes have been banned in many countries. The typical incubation (or "latency") period for bladder cancer in persons exposed to synthetic aniline dyes has been found to be about 18 to 22 years, which explains the typical 20-year lag between the start of chemical manufacture in a country and the first appearance of bladder cancer in workers.

Leukemia caused by occupational exposure to the solvent benzene was another early consequence of chemical manufacture. Like bladder cancer caused by synthetic aniline dyes, benzene-induced leukemia followed the chemical manufacturing industry as it spread internationally. Benzene has also been classified as a proven human carcinogen.

Asbestos exposure in World War II shipbuilders and in construction workers in countries around the world has been shown to be another cause of occupational cancer and is responsible for lung cancer and mesothelioma, a cancer of the lining of the lungs specific to asbestos exposure. Asbestos has been classified as a proven human carcinogen by the IARC.

Numerous synthetic chemicals, many of them still in wide use today, have been found to cause cancer in workers and are now classified by the IARC as either proven or probable human carcinogens. Other synthetic chemicals have been found to cause diseases of the brain and nervous system, reproductive system, endocrine organs, and immune systems of chemical workers.

Chemical workers have been described as "canaries in the coal mine", and disease in chemical workers often provides the first warning of future health problems in children.

How many untested chemicals are in commercial production today?

Since the 1940s, the volume and diversity of chemical production have both increased exponentially, as illustrated by Figure 2-1. During this time, more than 85,000 new synthetic chemicals have been invented and are registered today with the US Environmental Protection Agency (EPA). An even larger number of chemicals are registered internationally through

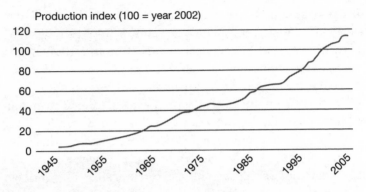

Figure 2-1 Chemical Production, United States, 1947–2007

the Organisation for Economic Cooperation and Development (OECD). These chemicals are used today in millions of consumer products, ranging from foods and food packaging to clothing, building materials, cleaning products, cosmetics, toys, and baby bottles.

The EPA has identified 3,000 synthetic chemicals as "high-production-volume" chemicals, which are defined as chemicals produced or imported in quantities of more than a million pounds per year. They are the chemicals that are in widest use and therefore have the greatest potential for dissemination in the environment and for human exposure. These chemicals are found today in air, food, and drinking water around the world.

Have some manufactured chemicals benefited children's health?

Very definitely, yes! Some new chemicals have profoundly benefited children's health. Antibiotics have helped control the major communicable diseases. Drinking water disinfectants have reduced deaths from dysentery. Chemotherapy agents have made possible the cure of many childhood cancers. Chemicals are central to modern construction and transportation systems. They are an essential building block of daily life.

But other new synthetic chemicals have been responsible for episodes of disease, death, and environmental degradation. Many of these episodes have resulted in severe injury to children.

A fundamental problem is that often little or no assessment is made of the safety or potential toxicity of new chemicals before they are brought to market. This failure to exercise due diligence makes it impossible to know which chemicals will be beneficial and which need to be treated with caution. It also sets the stage for potential health problems.

How are new chemicals developed and brought to market?

The short answer: With great enthusiasm, but without much regulation or vetting for health implications.

New chemicals are typically brought to market with great fanfare, come rapidly into widespread use in industrial settings and consumer products, and then become widely disseminated in the environment. After years or even decades, some materials that were initially hailed as beneficial have been found to have harmful effects on children's health and the environment—dangers that were neither considered nor even imagined before their introduction.

A recurrent theme in these episodes has been that commercial introduction of new chemicals has time and again preceded any prudent effort to assess their safety or toxicity—in particular, any efforts to examine impacts on human health. Historical examples of substances that were introduced with great fanfare, inadequately tested for safety or toxicity, and belatedly found to have caused great harm to human health and the environment include: the addition of lead to paint and gasoline; the use of asbestos for insulation and fireproofing products; the use of DDT as a pesticide; the introduction of thalidomide as a nausea-control agent in pregnancy; the widespread use of polychlorinated biphenyls (PCBs) in electrical transformers; the use of the synthetic hormone diethylstilbestrol (DES) to prevent miscarriage in pregnancy; and the use of ozone-destroying chlorofluorocarbons (CFCs) in refrigeration units.

This sequence of events has already been repeated in the 21st century, with new chemicals added to plastics and other consumer products. Two types of plastics additives—phthalates and bisphenol A (BPA)—have both been implicated in disruption of normal childhood development. Brominated flame retardants placed into couches, carpets, mattresses, and computers have been shown to cause delays in brain development with loss of IQ points. Organophosphate insecticides have been shown to cause microcephaly, a smaller than normal head that is linked to reduced brain size, as well as delayed development and behavioral problems. (Each of these topics is discussed in greater detail in other chapters of this book.)

Initially, all of these chemicals were deemed safe in the absence of any detailed examination before subsequently being found to cause disease in children.

Have there been there early warnings of chemical problems?

Yes. Increased rates of chemical-related diseases and disorders have been one early warning of new chemical hazards. A second warning has been seen in the effects of man-made chemicals on the environment.

The environmental effects of toxic chemicals were first brought to widespread attention through the publication in 1962 of *Silent Spring*, an iconic book by biologist Rachel Carson. *Silent Spring* detailed the dangers of pesticides to wildlife, specifically the role of the insecticide DDT in nearly causing the extinction of the osprey and the American bald eagle. It ushered in the environmental movement in the United States. Carson's book was hailed by scientists and the media but criticized by the chemical industry. It has become a classic and contributed to the formation of the EPA and to the federal ban on commercial production of the pesticide DDT.

Concerns about the effects of chemicals on the endocrine systems of wildlife and people that Rachel Carson had noted in *Silent Spring* were voiced again in 1996 in *Our Stolen Future: Are We Threatening Our Fertility, Intelligence, and Survival? A Scientific Detective Story* a book by Theo Colborn and colleagues, who coined the term *endocrine disruptors* to describe how manufactured chemicals could mimic the actions of natural hormones in wildlife and in people.

In some instances, industries with deeply vested interests in protecting markets for hazardous chemicals—such as the lead, tobacco, asbestos, and pesticide production industries—have actively opposed efforts to understand and control children's exposures to these materials. These industries have used highly sophisticated disinformation campaigns to confuse the public and discredit science. Lobbyists and scientists in the pay of the industries have attacked the expertise and claims of pediatricians, researchers, and environmental scientists who called attention to the risks of emerging technologies and new chemicals, just as they did in previous decades in the case of lead and mercury. Today, industry-sponsored disinformation campaigns are active around chlorinated solvents, organophosphate pesticides, and chemical herbicides.

How many of today's chemicals have been tested for safety or toxicity?

The majority of the 3,000 high-production-volume chemicals have not undergone even minimal assessment for safety or potential toxicity. Only approximately 20% of high-production-volume chemicals have been screened for their potential to disrupt early human development or to cause disease in infants and children. Accordingly, we have no knowledge of the possible dangers to children of most of the synthetic chemicals in the world today.

Even less is known about the potential effects of children's simultaneous exposure to multiple chemicals, or about how chemicals may interact with one another in the human body, possibly causing synergistic adverse effects on health.

Why have chemicals not been tested for safety or toxicity?

For decades, the chemical industry has hampered efforts in Congress and in EPA to achieve effective regulation of chemical substances known or suspected to be harmful to children's health. The failure of the Toxic Substances Control Act (TSCA), a 1976 law intended to promote testing of new and existing chemicals for potential toxicity, was the result of such interference. The legislation never achieved its goal because within one year of its passage into law, a decision was made to "grandfather in"—and presume safe—the 62,000 chemicals that were already on the market, without any requirement for toxicity testing. These chemicals were allowed to remain in commerce unless EPA made a definitive finding that the chemical posed an "unreasonable risk to human health or to the environment."

The "unreasonable risk" standard has been a major barrier to the regulation of industrial and consumer chemicals. Because TCSA places the burden of proof on the EPA to prove harm after a chemical has been released, rather than on chemical manufacturers before the release of a chemical, nearly all of the untested chemicals remain in the market. The EPA has been able to remove chemicals from the market only when a lengthy process shows there is overwhelming evidence of potential harm. As a result, only five chemicals have been controlled under the TCSA in the nearly 40 years since its passage. These chemicals are polychlorinated biphenyls (PCBs), chlorofluorocarbons, dioxin, asbestos, and hexavalent chromium.

What is the Safe Chemicals Act?

The Safe Chemicals Act was legislation initially proposed by the late Senator Frank Lautenberg (D-NJ) to revamp TSCA more than a decade before his death in 2013. Lautenberg's legislation had bounced around in Congressional committees and in various stages of revision for a decade, all the while facing opposition from both the chemical industry and members of Congress with ties to the industry.

In June 2016, the United States passed new legislation to revamp TSCA. The new law—the Frank R. Lautenberg Chemical Safety for the 21st Century Act—requires that the EPA assess the safety of any new chemical before it is allowed to enter the market, to prioritize and test the safety of existing chemicals, and to evaluate the safety of chemicals using a standard that considers only hazards to health and the environment and does not consider the costs of protective action. This law was supported by members of both parties. It was enacted after many years of effort by public health and environmental groups and public-interest lawyers, and despite relentless opposition by industry groups. In spite of some shortcomings, it is one of the strongest environmental laws enacted in the United States. While its implementation will require much logistical work by the EPA—an agency that faces redirection and cutbacks in the Donald J. Trump administration—it represents a seismic change in the landscape of chemicals, environment, and human health.

In December 2016, the EPA released its list of the first ten chemicals to be reviewed under new legislation (see Table 2-1).

The history and failure of the Toxic Substances Control Act are a cautionary tale for the new law. Its efficacy will be largely determined by the courage and integrity of the elected officials and EPA scientists charged with instituting and enforcing it.

What are countries outside of the United States doing to promote chemical safety?

Approaches to managing children's exposure to chemicals vary from country to country. The European Union has gone to the greatest lengths to promote chemical safety, passing a law called the Registration, Evaluation, Authorization and

Table 2-1 EPA's first ten chemicals for review under the Lautenberg Chemical Safety Act

Chemical	Uses/Locations	Health/Environmental Effects
1,4-dioxane	Groundwater pollutant; possible contaminant of many cosmetics, cleaners.	Possible human carcinogen.
1-bromopropane	Aerosol spray adhesives, aerosol spot removers, aerosol cleaners/degreasers.	National Toxicology Program classifies it as "reasonably anticipated to be a human carcinogen." Reproductive and developmental effects.
Asbestos	Occasionally found in auto brake pads and clutches, vinyl tiles, roofing materials and children's toys made with talc.	Known carcinogen, causes fatal lung disease (asbestosis).
Carbon tetrachloride	Solvent. Used to manufacture industrial chemicals. No longer used in consumer products.	Probable human carcinogen. Toxic to liver and kidneys; may harm the central nervous system.
HBCD (hexabromocyclododecane; cyclic aliphatic bromide cluster)	Flame retardant used primarily in rigid polystyrene house insulation. Can also contaminate food and dust.	Highly persistent and bioaccumulative in the environment, and highly toxic to aquatic organisms. HBCD harms human reproduction and development.
Methylene chloride	Paint stripping, vapor degreasing, printing, foam manufacturing, spice extraction, electronics manufacturing, chemical manufacturing, cleaning.	Probable human carcinogen.
NMP (N-methylpyrrolidone)	Paint stripping.	Reproductive toxicant.
Pigment Violet 29	Industrial colorant used in plastic and coatings. The EPA says it is "widely used in consumer products," but specific uses are not clear. Approved as an indirect food active.	Persistent in the environment and toxic to aquatic organisms.
PERC (perchloroethylene, tetrachloroethylene)	Dry cleaning, groundwater contamination.	Likely to be carcinogenic to humans; toxic to the nervous system
TCE (trichloroethyiene)	Dry cleaning, industrial uses, and a handful of consumer products for arts and crafts, auto products, home maintenance and home offices.	Carcinogenic to humans; toxic to the nervous system.

Source: EPA list of chemicals for review. Available at www.epa.gov/assessing-and-managing-chemicals-under-tsca/evaluating-risk-existing-chemicals-under-tsca

Restriction of Chemical Substances Act (REACH) in 2007. REACH requires the chemical industry to conduct extensive safety testing of new chemicals before the chemicals are allowed to come to market. Companies must submit their testing information to the European Chemical Agency, which in turn uses the information to determine whether it is safe to allow a chemical to enter consumer products and to craft regulations that protect the health of children. Under REACH, hazardous chemicals that are still allowed in consumer products in the United States have been banned in Europe. The European Chemical Agency is also developing a public database that will make information on hazardous chemicals widely accessible to the general public.

Following the lead of the European Union, a number of countries (including Japan, Norway, Mexico, Argentina, and Australia) are now looking more closely at the potential harm a chemical may cause before permitting it to enter markets. If there is not enough scientific evidence to ensure that a chemical will not harm a child's development, the substance is banned in those countries.

What is the impact of REACH, the European chemical safety law, on children in the United States?

An unexpected consequence of the passage of REACH and other similarly strong safety laws in countries outside of the United States is that, while children in those countries are protected from toxic chemicals, children in the United States continue to be exposed.

Some of this difference is attributable to lax legislation in the United States, specifically the now defunct Toxic Substances Control Act described in the preceding section. But there is also a market component: when chemicals are rejected for sale in the European Union, the chemical manufacturers divert the banned chemicals to countries with less rigid standards.

In effect, the United States has become one of the "dumping grounds" for products deemed unsafe by Europe.

Improved safety for children in the United States is within reach. Multinational companies already produce the healthier products that meet the stringent regulations of the European Union, so even while their unsafe products remain available in the United States, they don't have to be. The safer products— phthalate-free toys, cadmium-free computer parts, electronics that do not contain brominated flame retardants, and cosmetics that do not contain phthalates, lead, or other toxic chemicals— are available through tighter regulation.

It is to be hoped that the Lautenberg Chemical Safety Act will close the current loopholes in protection for American children, but only time will tell.

How do we know that children are being exposed to untested chemicals in the environment?

We know that children are exposed to untested chemicals because in regular national surveys conducted by the Centers for Disease Control and Prevention (CDC), measurable quantities of 200 high-production-volume chemicals have been detected in the blood and urine of virtually all US residents, including pregnant women. While these measured levels are generally low, they are much higher than the levels of the same chemicals that would have been found in the bodies of most Americans one or two generations earlier.

Untested chemicals are also routinely detected today in the breast milk of nursing mothers and in the umbilical cord blood of newborn infants.

What are the dangers of failure to test chemicals for safety and toxicity?

The absence of information about the possible hazards of chemicals in wide use is fraught with risk. Unless studies are conducted to specifically seek harmful effects associated with chemical exposures, silent injury to children's health can go unrecognized for years, or even decades. The risk inherent in the long-standing failure to test chemicals for safety has produced devastating results, among them the "silent epidemic" of childhood lead poisoning that affected children in the United States and around the world throughout much of the 20th century.

In the silent epidemic of childhood lead poisoning, millions of American children were exposed to excessive levels of lead from the 1920s to the early 1980s. The major sources of exposure were lead added to gasoline to improve engine performance and lead-based paint. Many thousands of children born in those years suffered low-level lead poisoning, which typically has no symptoms (and thus is called a silent disease). Lead caused brain injury in thousands of American children and was diagnosed by loss of IQ points, shortening of attention span, and disruption of behavior. Children who suffered low-grade lead poisoning with brain damage were more likely than other children of their generation to be dyslexic, to drop out of school, to engage in delinquent and criminal behavior, and ultimately to be incarcerated.

The story of the lead poisoning epidemic is a warning. It shows us that low-grade exposures to toxic chemicals can cause real damage to children and have real costs for our society. Our children pay a high price for our failure to require the testing of all chemicals.

A similar slow-motion tragedy is playing out today in the case of brominated flame retardants. Brominated flame retardants are synthetic chemicals that, since the 1970s, have been added to furniture, carpets, computers, mattresses, and even children's clothing. Use of brominated flame retardants is increasing worldwide.

The problem is that the brominated flame retardants do not remain in the consumer products to which they are added. They escape from these products, get into house dust, onto children's hands, and into food. Human exposure is widespread. National surveys conducted by the CDC show that virtually all Americans of all ages, including young children and pregnant women, have measurable levels of brominated flame retardants in their bodies. Brominated flame retardants concentrate to especially high levels in human breast milk. Within the past few years, high-quality studies have shown that babies exposed in their mother's womb to brominated flame retardants have lower IQs, shortened attention spans, and persistent behavioral problems. These problems persist at least until age 7 years, and they may well last lifelong. Legislative efforts to control the use of brominated flame retardants are just beginning, and these efforts are being fiercely resisted by the chemical industry. Yet despite this opposition, more than a dozen states including California, Oregon, Idaho, Illinois, Michigan, and Vermont have now passed policies banning these chemicals.

Speaking on the failure to test chemicals for safety and toxicity, the late Herbert L. Needleman, a noted pediatrician and pioneer in the study of childhood lead poisoning, observed, "We are conducting a massive toxicological experiment in the world today, and our children and grandchildren are the unknowing, unconsenting subjects."

Are there other chemicals in wide use today that are harming children's health?

Very likely. Based on the large number of chemicals currently in production and the failure to test most of them for safety and toxicity, the likelihood is high that certain chemicals in wide use today are causing silent injury to infants and children and that their toxicity has not yet been discovered.

The problem of children's exposure to untested chemicals is shown in Figure 2-2—the "chemical iceberg."

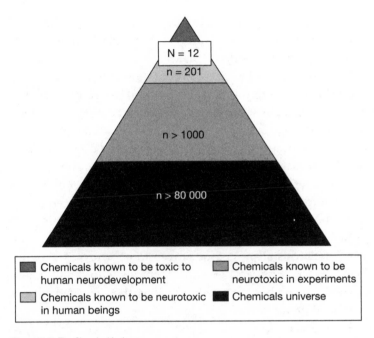

Figure 2-2 The Chemical Iceberg

Grandjean, P, Landrigan PJ, Developmental Neurotoxicity of Industrial Chemicals: a Silent Pandemic. Lancet 2006;368:2167-78.

In the diagram of the chemical iceberg, n refers to the number of chemicals in each slice of the triangle, and the key shows what is known about those chemicals.

At the tip of the iceberg are about a dozen chemicals now definitely linked to developmental disorders of the brain and other organs in children. These chemicals are known with certainty to cause lowered IQ, behavioral disorders, attention deficit/hyperactivity disorder, and autism spectrum disorders. Painstaking medical research has pieced together each of the complex puzzles linking these chemicals role to developmental abnormalities in children.

Yet, although exposures to these chemicals now form a clear and recognizable picture, generations of children have been, and continue to be, exposed to lead, mercury, PCBs, pesticides, polycyclic aromatic hydrocarbons, brominated flame retardants, bisphenol A, and phthalates.

The next largest piece of the iceberg shows the approximately 200 industrial chemicals that are known to be neurotoxicants—chemicals capable of damaging the brain and nervous system. Studies in industrial settings have found these chemicals to be toxic to the brains of adult workers exposed occupationally. Each of these chemicals was identified as neurotoxic when it caused serious, clinically obvious, acute effects in workers exposed to it in the industrial workplace, yet the potential for these chemicals to injure children has never been examined.

The next lower layer of the iceberg shows that there are 1,000 chemicals suspected or proven to be neurotoxic in animals. Again, although these are chemicals with a high likelihood of causing human health problems, they have never been examined in humans of any age.

In summary, there are at least 1,200 consumer and industrial chemicals at large in the world today with the potential to cause damage to children's developing brains and nervous systems whose toxicity to children has never been examined.

The largest portion of the iceberg shows the more than 80,000 new synthetic chemicals that have been produced during the past 50 years. Little is known about the toxicity of most of these chemicals. Yet children are exposed to unknown numbers of them every day.

If nothing is done, is it likely that this problem will continue to grow?

Yes. The problem of chemical exposure continues to grow in the United States and in other countries around the world. New chemicals are introduced every month and global production of manufactured chemicals is increasing at a rate of over 3% per year.

Today, with the globalization of trade, chemical manufacture is shifting increasingly to developing countries, where labor costs are low and often there are few environmental and public health protections. Chemical pollution is increasing in developing nations, and hazardous wastes are accumulating. These trends may be expected to accelerate in the years ahead.

At the same time, pollution-related noncommunicable diseases, such as asthma, heart disease, stroke, and cancer are becoming epidemic in countries where they were previously seldom seen. The once separate patterns of disease in developed and developing countries are converging.

3

CHILDREN'S UNIQUE VULNERABILITY TO TOXIC CHEMICALS IN THE ENVIRONMENT

Are children more vulnerable than adults to toxic chemicals in the environment?

Children are far more sensitive to toxic chemicals than adults. This sensitivity reflects the combination of children's disproportionately greater exposures plus their exquisite biological sensitivity.

What historical evidence supports the argument that children are vulnerable to toxic chemicals in the environment?

Two tragic episodes—the thalidomide epidemic in Europe in the 1950s and 1960s and the DES epidemic in the United States in the 1960s and 70s—were watershed events that led to wide recognition of children's exquisite sensitivity to toxic chemicals.

Thalidomide is a synthetic chemical that was developed in the 1950s. It is a sedative that was found to be effective in controlling morning sickness during the first trimester of pregnancy, and it was prescribed to women early in pregnancy to alleviate nausea and vomiting. Most use of the drug's use occurred in Europe.

Within a year after the initial use of thalidomide to control morning sickness, pediatricians in Europe began to observe increasing numbers of babies born with a previously rare birth defect of the limbs called phocomelia—a congenital malformation in which the child's limbs, usually the arms, are extremely short or missing. Virtually all of the affected babies had been exposed in the womb to thalidomide. Thalidomide's effects were found to be most harmful when it was taken between days 34 and 50 of pregnancy, which is precisely the stage in which limbs are forming.

In addition to interfering with limb formation, thalidomide was also associated with deformed eyes, ears, hearts, alimentary tracts, and urinary tracts; it also produced blindness, deafness, and increased risk of autism. The pattern of the abnormalities reflected the exact timing of exposure, because different organs in a baby are formed at different times during pregnancy.

Thalidomide was never licensed in the United States, thanks to the watchfulness of Dr. Frances Kelsey, a physician working for the US Food and Drug Administration, who had concerns based on the drug's performance in animal testing studies. The medication was nonetheless prescribed extensively to pregnant women around the world, and more than 10,000 cases of phocomelia were reported (including 8,000 in Germany alone) before thalidomide was removed from the market and the epidemic was halted. Mothers who took the medication were physically unaffected.

The second tragedy involved diethylstilbestrol (DES), a synthetic form of estrogen developed in the 1940s. It was prescribed to as many as five million pregnant women in the United States in the 1960s and early 1970s to block spontaneous abortions (miscarriages) and to promote fetal growth. A decade later, gynecologists began observing cases of a rare cancer, adenocarcinoma of the vagina, in young women. Peak incidence of the cancer occurred in the years immediately after puberty.

Careful medical detective work revealed that the great majority of the young women with vaginal cancer had been exposed to DES in their mothers' wombs. Their mothers were physically unaffected. Further long-term follow-up studies have now shown that after age 40, DES daughters have a 2.5-fold increased incidence of breast cancer. Reproductive abnormalities have also been seen in DES sons.

The thalidomide and DES tragedies demonstrated with painful clarity that infants and children, especially during the nine months before birth, are much more sensitive than adults to toxic chemicals in the environment and can suffer unique forms of injury that have no counterparts in adult life. Furthermore, before the thalidomide and DES tragedies, it was widely believed that the placenta formed an inviolable barrier that protected the fetus against toxic chemicals. That belief is now understood to be untrue, because these events proved that toxic chemicals can cross the placenta into the body of the unborn child.

Why are infants and children so sensitive to toxic chemicals?

Research undertaken in the years following the thalidomide and DES tragedies identified important differences in patterns of exposure and in sensitivity between children and adults that account for children's susceptibility to toxic chemicals.

Much of the knowledge in this area was codified in a 1993 report by the US National Academy of Sciences (NAS) titled *Pesticides in the Diets of Infants and Children*. The analysis was commissioned by the Committee on Agriculture of the US Senate, and it was triggered by rising concern about children's exposures to toxic and possibly cancer-causing pesticides in fruits and vegetables. The report found four critical differences between children and adults that account for children's vulnerability to toxic chemicals:

- **Children experience greater exposure than adults based on their body size.**
  Children have disproportionately large intakes of air, food, and water. Infants, for example, have respiratory

rates that are twice as great as those of adults. Pound per pound of body weight, they inhale twice as much air. Thus, they are at increased risk of absorbing airborne toxins. Likewise, children eat more food and drink much more water per pound of body weight than adults. Children take in three to four times more calories per pound than adults, and a 6-month-old infant drinks seven times more water per pound of body weight than an adult.

The differences between children and adults in dietary exposure become especially striking when you consider their actual diets. Some children consume extraordinary amounts of certain foods, such as milk, juices, and fruits, for certain periods of time in early infancy and childhood. If those foods happen to be contaminated with high levels of pesticides, and, worse yet, if they are contaminated by multiple pesticides, the cumulative dose delivered to the children can be quite large.

Another difference between children and adults is that children have a larger surface-to-volume ratio and more permeable skin, two factors that lead to greater skin absorption of toxic chemicals.

Children's behaviors further exacerbate their intake of toxic chemicals. Most children actively explore their environments, and young children frequently put things in their mouth, including hands and things they pick up and examine. This normal oral exploratory behavior can lead to significant ingestion of toxic substances.

Children also spend their time in different physical locations than adults, and these differences can increase their exposures. Infants and young children spend much of their time on the floor. They are therefore at disproportionate risk of exposure to house dust that may be contaminated with lead, brominated flame retardants, or pesticides. Toddlers, because of their short stature, breathe air that is much closer to the ground than that inhaled by adults. They are therefore at increased risk of inhaling vapors of solvents or pesticides that may form layers near the floor. In addition, children are exposed to preschool or school classroom environments and playgrounds. Schools and playgrounds are too often built on relatively undesirable lands and the facilities may be old, poorly maintained, and poorly ventilated.

- **Children's metabolic pathways are immature.**
  Children's ability to break down and excrete toxic chemicals is different from that of adults. In some instances, infants are actually at lower risk of injury by toxic chemicals because they cannot convert the chemicals to their active forms. But in many more cases, children are more vulnerable, because they are less able than adults to detoxify and excrete toxic compounds. As a result, many toxic chemicals spend more time in the child's body before being excreted.

  For example, studies show that the adult body can reduce the blood level of one common pesticide (chlorpyrifos, an organophosphate pesticide used around lawns and gardens) by half in 6 hours, but it takes an infant 36 hours to do the same thing. That gives the toxic pesticide six times longer to harm the infant's body.

- **Children are undergoing rapid growth and development, and their delicate developmental processes are easily disrupted.**
  Children have exquisitely complex and delicate developmental processes. These processes have been compared to a complex symphony in which each instrument has to play the correct note at precisely the right moment or the result is chaos. The processes are orchestrated with clockwork precision during the nine months of pregnancy. They continue after birth, through early childhood, and even into adolescence and adult life (Figure 3-1).

During the nine months of pregnancy, the orchestra is playing at a dizzying pace. Each minute, each hour, and each day

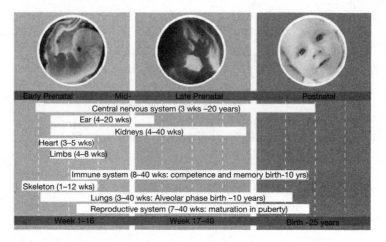

Figure 3-1 Stages of Human Development

Courtesy of Dr Jerrold Heindel, US National Institute of Environmental Health Science.

produce major, noticeable changes in the developing baby. In order for a child to develop normally, predictable events must occur at very specific times. Cells multiply and move in a complicated dance pattern to form the brain and nervous system and to develop the arms, legs, and facial features. At the same time, other cells are moving to form and develop internal organs, the immune system, and the reproductive organs.

All of these fast-moving changes are closely controlled by natural hormones. Hormones are powerful chemicals secreted in minute amounts by the endocrine glands in the body—the pituitary gland, the thyroid, the adrenal glands, the ovaries, and the testicles. Hormones are signaling chemicals. They direct cells in the body to turn switches on and off, to go fast or to slow down. Hormones regulate growth and development in infants and children, reproduction in young adults, and aging in older adults. The network of hormones in the human body is called the endocrine system. Think of the endocrine system as a complex computer in which messages are transmitted between cells via chemical messengers rather than via electrical signals.

A child's development does not stop at birth. During infancy, childhood, and puberty, equally complex growth and development occur. The continuum of rapid development is now quite visible as the infant grows into a young child, developing new abilities and behaviors almost daily! The very definition of childhood implies a rate of change and development not ever experienced again at any time in life.

Like the conductor of the orchestra wielding his baton, the endocrine system releases its natural hormones at precise points in time to tell the body what to do next throughout childhood and into early adulthood. At times, especially during early childhood, the orchestra is playing at breakneck speed. In later childhood, its pace is slower, only to speed up again as the teen years approach. Ultimately, the orchestral symphony of child development reaches its final chords with the emergence of the young adult.

This great complexity of early human development creates *windows of vulnerability*, periods of heightened sensitivity to toxic chemicals that exist only in early life and have no counterpart in adulthood.

Most of the windows of vulnerability occur during the nine months of pregnancy, and others occur during early childhood. Exposures to even minute quantities of toxic chemicals during these sensitive periods—levels that would have no adverse effect on an adult—can lead to permanent injury to the brain, reproductive organs, immune system, and other organ systems.

Children have more future years of life than do most adults, with more time to develop noncommunicable diseases that may have been triggered by early environmental exposure.

Compared with adults, children have many more years ahead of them. This means that children have a much longer period of time in which to develop disease that is caused by early-life exposures to toxic chemicals. Many diseases triggered by toxic chemicals, such as cancer and brain diseases, are now understood to evolve over the course of many years or even decades. This time is termed an *incubation period* or latency period. Some of the neurological diseases, such as Parkinson's disease, and certain cancers are now suspected of having links with early exposures to toxic chemicals in the environment, even exposures in the womb.

On the basis of its analysis of children's sensitivity to toxic chemicals, the National Academy of Sciences Committee on Pesticides in the Diets of Infants and Children concluded in their 1993 report that the laws and regulations then in force in the United States were not adequately protecting children against pesticides and other toxic chemicals. The Committee recommended fundamental revamping of US pesticide law to better protect children's health.

What changes in public policy resulted from the NAS Pesticides in the Diets of Infants and Children *report?*

The National Academy of Sciences (NAS) report *Pesticides in the Diets of Infants and Children* catalyzed a profound shift in public policy, first in the United States and then globally. The report's oft-quoted conclusion was that "children are not little adults." This concise takeaway raised the previously overlooked issue of children's sensitivity to toxic chemicals to the highest levels of national policy.

Prior to publication of the NAS report, virtually all research in toxicology and all risk assessment and policy formulation in environmental health in the United States had focused on protecting the average adult. That research did not take into account the unique exposures or the special susceptibilities of fetuses, infants, and children.

The old approach to regulation of pesticides is a good example. Prior to publication of the NAS report, the levels of pesticides, termed *tolerance levels*, that were permitted on fruits and vegetables sold in markets were set at levels considered to be safe for adults.

However, there were two shortcomings with this approach. First, the old pesticide tolerance levels were not health-based. Instead they tried to balance the protection of human health against the costs of regulation. Often, the scales tipped against the health of the public. The second, and even more serious, shortcoming was that the older regulations paid no attention to the unique exposures or special susceptibilities of infants and children. They assumed that the population was comprised solely of adults and that a single tolerance level would protect people of all ages against pesticides in agricultural products.

The NAS report fundamentally changed that. It gave lawmakers a new way of looking at the hazards of pesticides and other toxic chemicals. It provided the intellectual foundation for the Food Quality Protection Act of 1996, the US law governing use of pesticides and the first such statute in the United States to contain explicit provisions for the protection of children. Quite amazingly, the law was passed in 1996 by unanimous vote of both houses of the US Congress, and was signed into law by President Bill Clinton.

What has happened in the two decades since release of the NAS report Pesticides in the Diets of Infants and Children?

Over the two decades that have passed since publication of the NAS report and passage of the Food Quality Protection Act, research in children's environmental health has grown exponentially and has become an increasingly visible and important area of pediatrics. Dramatic increases in knowledge and understanding have resulted. Much of what has been learned since that time forms the basis of this book. But despite these gains in knowledge, children will continue be exposed to toxic chemicals in the environment on a daily basis until EPA and the Congress translate this knowledge into protective action.

What are international agencies doing about children's environmental health?

In 1997, the eight leading economic nations, the G8, issued a declaration at a meeting in Miami supporting the protection of children from health threats in the environment. All eight countries—the United States, Canada, Great Britain, France, Germany, Italy, Japan, and Russia—agreed in the Miami Declaration to make the protection of children's health against environmental threats a national priority.

Is the World Health Organization involved in protecting children against environmental threats to health?

The World Health Organization (WHO) has become deeply engaged in protecting children against environmental threats to health. In 1999, under the charismatic leadership of the late Dr. Jenny Pronczuk de Garbino, a WHO physician originally from Uruguay, WHO established the Task Force for the Protection of Children's Environmental Health.

The goal of the WHO task force has been to examine trends in pediatric disease and in the environment and to develop evidence-based strategies to prevent disease and disability associated with chemical and physical hazards.

A major finding that emerged from the work of the WHO task force is that chemical, physical, and biological hazards in the environment are responsible for 23% of deaths worldwide and for 26% of all deaths in children under the age of 5 years. This powerful conclusion continues to shape global health policy to this day.

The WHO has published important reports documenting in detail the impacts of unhealthy environments on children's health. The most recent of these reports, *Inheriting a Sustainable World: Atlas on Children's Health and the Environment*, was published in 2017.

4

THE LINKS BETWEEN TOXIC CHEMICALS IN THE ENVIRONMENT AND DISEASE IN CHILDREN

In recent decades, enormous growth has occurred in knowledge about the connections between toxic chemicals in the environment and disease in children, and this powerful body of medical and scientific evidence continues to grow. New discoveries of links between chemical exposures and childhood diseases are now reported almost monthly.

This chapter tells the story of how these discoveries were made. It summarizes what we know today about the connections between childhood diseases and toxic chemicals, describes the likely future direction of research in children's environmental health—the new branch of pediatrics that studies the impact of the environment on health and disease in children—and summarizes what parents need to know about the links between toxic chemicals and childhood disease.

What caused the recent surge in research into the effects of toxic chemicals on children's health?

Two driving forces have been responsible for this era of scientific discovery. The first is the National Academy of Science

(NAS) report, *Pesticides in the Diets of Infants and Children*, published in 1993. Publication of this report coupled with the passage in 1996 of the Food Quality Protection Act, described in Chapter 3, made the protection of children against environmental hazards a national priority in the United States and spurred increases in research on the connections between children's health and toxic chemicals. This research has identified previously unsuspected environmental causes of disease in children. These research findings have guided successful disease prevention programs and have greatly increased interest in environmental threats to children's health among students, parents, teachers, elected officials, policymakers, and the general public.

The second driving force has been the alarming increase in noncommunicable diseases in children over the past 3 decades—asthma, cancer, autism, attention deficit/hyperactivity disorder (ADHD), birth defects, obesity, and diabetes—as described in Chapter 2.

Scientific advances in five areas have been especially important for increasing knowledge about how toxic chemicals cause disease in children:

1. The realization that chemical toxicity can occur in children with minimal or no symptoms—subclinical toxicity
2. Understanding the societal implications of subclinical toxicity
3. Stronger epidemiological studies based on advances in exposure-measurement technology
4. Strong studies that have made use of new, sensitive biological markers of health outcomes
5. The decoding of the human genome, which has enabled scientists to better understand the impact of the environment on genes and to understand why different children have different individual susceptibilities to toxic chemicals.

Can a toxic chemical cause problems in children who show no symptoms or minimal symptoms?

Yes. *Subclinical toxicity* is the concept that toxic chemicals can cause health problems in children without producing any symptoms. Subclinical toxicity is also called silent toxicity. While subclinical poisoning does not cause obvious symptoms, its damage can be significant and can be observed on IQ tests, X-rays, lung function tests or other evaluations of children's health.

By contrast, when poisoning is caused by exposure to a high dose of a toxic chemical, the symptoms are severe and very obvious. Acute high-dose childhood lead poisoning produces profound symptoms such as seizures, brain damage and death. Severe, acute methylmercury poisoning causes profound mental retardation in children exposed in the womb. An episode of acute methylmercury poisoning occurred in Minimata, Japan, in the 1950s and 60s and caused profound mental retardation in children who were exposed *in utero* after their mothers ate fish from water contaminated by mercury waste from an industrial plant. Severe, high dose poisoning is like the tip of the iceberg—the small, visible part of something much bigger.

Subclinical toxicity is the much larger, less visible part of the iceberg that escapes notice until it is specifically sought out. Its subtle health problems can be missed by parents and they are not evident on a standard pediatric examination. Hence they are called subclinical. They can be found only through special testing, such as IQ testing or neurobehavioral assessment.

In the case of lead poisoning, subclinical toxicity was first recognized in the 1970s in studies of children exposed to lead. The largest and most important of the studies were directed by pediatrician and child psychiatrist Herbert L. Needleman. His meticulous clinical and epidemiological evaluations demonstrated that even very low levels of lead exposure that produce no obvious symptoms are nonetheless able to cause "silent" brain injury in children, resulting in a reduction in intelligence, shortening of attention span, and alteration of behavior.

Long-term follow-up of the children exposed to lead found that they went on to have elevated rates of reading difficulties, school failure, and incarceration. The studies by Needleman and others made it clear that subclinical toxicity with damage to the brain and nervous system can cause significant injury in children that lasts a lifetime.

Subclinical toxicity caused by methylmercury has been identified in infants exposed prenatally to methylmercury at levels too low to produce obvious symptoms. A study in New Zealand showed that children exposed to methylmercury prenatally had a 3-point decrease in IQ as well as alterations in their behavior. A large study of prenatally exposed children in the Faroe Islands of Denmark also found evidence that children had impairments in memory, attention, language, and visual-spatial perception. The severity of the impairments was directly related to the degree of exposure to methylmercury. Another study in the Seychelles Islands also showed some evidence of prenatal neurotoxicity. The US National Academy of Sciences reviewed these studies and concluded that there is now strong evidence showing methylmercury can damage an unborn child's brain and nervous system, even at low levels of exposure.

The concept of subclinical toxicity has now expanded well beyond lead and methylmercury to include a wide range of toxic chemicals that cause adverse effects in multiple organ systems in children. While subclinical effects may be small at the individual level, the aggregate effects at a population level can have far-reaching economic and is social consequences.

What is the impact of subclinical toxicity on society?

When subclinical or silent toxicity is widespread among children, it can have far-reaching social and economic consequences. Widespread exposures to toxic chemicals that damage the developing brain and nervous system are especially dangerous, because the damage caused by these chemicals is silent—it is not easily detected without knowing how to look for it. It is not identified by the usual health statistics kept by most countries and may continue unabated for a long time. Substantial damage to a society can result: it can increase the number of children who need special education services, and more children may have have attention deficit disorders and behavioral problems that limit their ability to fully contribute to society as adults.

The epidemic of childhood lead poisoning is a dramatic example. Millions of American children were exposed to excessive levels of lead from the 1920s to the early 1980s, when lead (in the form of tetraethyl lead) was routinely added to gasoline to increase engine performance. At peak use in the 1970s, annual consumption of tetraethyl lead in gasoline in the United States was nearly 100,000 tons. Virtually all of this lead was released into the environment through the exhaust pipes of cars and trucks. It caused extensive environmental contamination, especially within cities and along roadways. The average blood lead level of US children was close to 20 µg/dL.

Many thousands of children born in that era suffered unrecognized brain injury, with loss of IQ points, shortening of their attention span, and disruption of behavior as the result of their exposure to lead from gasoline. It is estimated that the epidemic of subclinical lead poisoning may have reduced the number of children with higher intelligence (IQ scores above 130 points) by over 50% and likewise caused a more than 50% increase in the number with IQ scores below 70 (see Figure 4-1). In the United States alone, the total number of children at risk of exposure to airborne lead during the 40 years of its use was approximately 100 million.

As a result of widespread exposure to lead, there was an increase in the number of children who did poorly in school, who required special education and other remedial programs, and who could not contribute fully to society when they

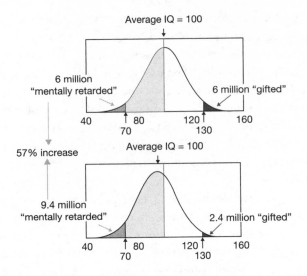

Figure 4-1 Intelligence losses associated with a 5-point drop in IQ of a pollution of 100 million children

With permission of Prof Bernard Weiss, University of Rochester.

became adults. At the same time, there was a reduction in the number of children with higher intelligence scores.

Damage to a society by toxic chemicals can be catastrophic, and has been so throughout history. Some historians have speculated that the fall of the Roman Empire may have been caused by widespread lead poisoning. It is known that the Romans used lead, which is a very soft metal, to line the aqueducts carrying water from the mountains to their towns. Roman citizens' exposure to lead in their water supply may have caused a loss of intelligence and diminished fertility, especially among the upper classes, who also used a special concoction of lead to sweeten their wine.

What research methods are used to identify links between chemical exposure and childhood disease?

To find links between childhood disease and exposure to a toxic chemical, researchers need accurate measurements of exposures and of disease. New research methods in epidemiology (the study of diseases in populations) are being used to study how populations of children are affected by exposures to toxic chemicals.

A standard epidemiological research design called a prospective birth cohort study enrolls pregnant women, and the researchers measure the environmental exposures that the women have during their pregnancy and then study the health of the women's children throughout their childhood and beyond. Prospective birth cohort studies are typically very large, with many women enrolled. Children in the studies receive periodic follow-up examinations, sometimes over many years.

Prospective birth cohort studies have become much more powerful tools for the scientific discovery of environmental causes of disease in children due to advances in technology. Today, if a researcher is doing a study involving indoor air pollution, for example, the researcher no longer needs to develop estimates of air pollution at different times of the day by using statistical models. Instead, the researcher can accurately measure a woman's actual exposure to air pollution throughout her pregnancy using a highly sophisticated, portable air sampler in a backpack to collect samples of the air in her apartment. In the same way, exposures during pregnancy to other toxic chemicals, such as lead, secondhand cigarette smoke, or pesticides, can be measured. A great strength of prospective study is that it permits real-time assessment of a woman's environmental exposures, months or years before any health effect might be noticed in her child. To establish the link between an environmental exposure and a childhood disease, it is no longer necessary for researchers to rely on the mother's memory of her past exposures.

The technology of exposure science has now expanded to the point that laboratory tests can accurately measure a person's exposure to environmental chemicals by measuring the chemical or its metabolic products in blood or body fluids. With technology advances, it is also becoming possible to measure an individual's susceptibility to a toxic chemical. Scientists studying the causes of disease have a growing ability to examine the role of *gene–environment interactions* and to explore how an environmental exposure affects the human genome.

With these new tools, the pace of scientific discovery in environmental pediatrics, the study of the impact of environmental exposures on child health, has accelerated.

The increasing use of sophisticated prospective birth cohort studies has already generated information on a series of previously unrecognized associations between environmental exposures and disease in children. As the pace of knowledge about environmental exposures and childhood disease continues to increase, we can expect to see rapid definition of which toxic chemicals need to be removed from the environment to protect the health of our children.

What new tools are used in current research in children's environmental health?

When today's researchers are trying to determine whether an environmental chemical is causing a disease or disorder in children, they utilize two important new technological tools:

1. sensitive and reliable biological markers (biomarkers) of the disease that can detect the disease or disorder at an early or subclinical stage, and
2. sensitive and specific biomarkers of exposure to a given chemical or combination of chemicals.

What is a biomarker of a disease?

In the early years of the 20th century, when physicians first discovered acute lead poisoning in children, the biomarkers or biological signs of the disease were the symptoms of the disease. In that era, when children were exposed to much higher levels of lead than today, symptoms were readily apparent, including vomiting, cramping, mental disruption, convulsions, and even death. The symptoms were clear indicators of lead poisoning.

In the 1960s and 1970s, when researchers identified subclinical lead poisoning at lower levels of exposure, they relied on more subtle biomarkers, such as blood lead levels, IQ tests, and nerve conduction studies, to make the diagnosis.

Today's sophisticated technology allows detection of biomarkers of disease that are tiny but measurable biochemical changes in children's bodies, or disruptions within cells (epigenetic changes), or disruptions of the genes (genetic mutations).

One example of the new sensitive and reliable biomarkers available with today's technology is a laboratory test that shows if a woman had become pregnant but had lost the developing embryo within a few hours, days, or weeks—even before she was aware she was pregnant. Another example of biomarker detection is pulmonary function testing to diagnose subtle decreases in lung function related to children's exposure to air pollution.

What is an example of a biomarker of exposure to a toxic chemical?

When a toxic chemical enters the body, it often leaves a biochemical footprint. Today, very sophisticated tests for the footprints (biomarkers) of exposures to lead and other toxic chemicals have been developed.

As an example, it has been known for many decades that when lead enters the body, some of it is deposited in teeth and bones. Herbert Needleman, a pioneer in research on lead in the 20th century, enlisted the assistance of children in grade schools in the Boston area to donate their baby teeth, so that their cumulative exposure to lead over the first 6 or 7 years of their lives could be accurately determined. His research led to a very clear understanding of the subclinical effects of lead and to the realization that there is no safe level for lead exposure.

Today, new bioimaging technology is expanding upon this concept and is providing a wealth of important new data from teeth. Teeth have growth rings that are similar to the growth rings in trees, and during pregnancy and in early childhood a new ring is formed every day. In trees, each growth ring can give specific information about the environmental conditions during its growing season—whether the climate was wet or dry, how plentiful the food supply was, and so on. In a similar fashion, creative and talented researchers are finding that teeth can be "mined" to provide needed information about exposures to toxic chemicals during the prenatal period and beyond. Very exciting, precise techniques for extracting data from different areas of shed teeth are yielding substantial information about prenatal exposure to toxic chemicals like manganese and lead. Additional biomarkers of exposures should lead to an explosive growth in information about the links between toxic exposures in the prenatal and childhood years to childhood disease as well as to diseases in later life. (The Resources section lists links to a few of these research studies.)

Finally, researchers have developed techniques based on the ability to decode the human genome to show that a toxic chemical has actually affected genes responsible for a disease.

In a recently published study, researchers used highly sophisticated laboratory technology to show that pesticides and many other endocrine-disrupting chemicals discussed in this book preferentially target genes that have been linked to autism. (See Carter and Blizard, 2016, in Resources.) This study is just one of a large number of recent research investigations making important links between toxic chemicals and disorders like autism, neurodevelopmental problems, reproductive and endocrine system abnormalities, and others.

What childhood diseases are currently linked to toxic environmental exposures?

There are five areas of current concern regarding childhood disease and toxic environmental exposure: asthma and other respiratory diseases, childhood cancer, neurodevelopmental disorders, reproductive disorders and endocrine disruptors, and childhood obesity.

Asthma and Other Respiratory Diseases

Infants and children are highly sensitive to air pollution. A 5-year-old child inhales about 25 liters of air each hour and more than 600 liters per day, much more per pound of body weight than an adult. As a result, substantial quantities of inhaled pollutants can be deposited on the delicate membranes that line children's respiratory tracts and lungs. With their immature immune systems, children are also much more likely than adults to contract upper respiratory infections, which cause sneezing and runny noses. Their developing respiratory system and lung function are also compromised by both indoor and outdoor air pollution.

Children living downwind of a pollution sources, such as a polluted city streets, major highways, or factory smokestacks, are exposed daily to elevated levels of air pollution from these combustion sources. Weather systems moving across the country from west to east can carry a mix of pollutants from factories and agriculture, including heavy metals, toxic chemicals, and pesticides. Combustion of heavy oils (#4 and #6 heating oils) in furnaces is an additional source of urban air pollution.

Inner city air pollution is caused primarily by gasoline and diesel exhaust emissions from motor vehicles—cars, trucks, and buses. Fine particles of soot and irritating and toxic gases produced by combustion, when exposed to sunlight, react with oxygen to produce a toxic smog containing carbon monoxide, nitrogen oxides, sulfur dioxide, and ozone—all of which irritate the lungs and respiratory system.

During the steamy, hot, still days of summer, levels of airborne pollutants can be very high, especially during the daytime when ozone levels peak. As night falls, the ozone levels decrease, but the fine particulate pollution often remains. So the "bad air" can extend well into the night and during periods when other pollutants diminish. Some of the particles are small enough to penetrate deep into the lungs and can be transported into the blood, carrying a toxic mixture of sulfur oxides, heavy metals, and other noxious materials directly into children's bodies.

Indoor air pollution can contain high levels of cigarette smoke, as well as the combustion products of poorly ventilated household stoves, furnaces, and fireplaces. When a house is well ventilated, the levels of indoor air pollution approximate those of outdoor air pollution, but when a house is closed up for heating or air conditioning, the indoor air pollution levels rise, especially if there is a smoker in the house or a poorly ventilated stove or fireplace.

Exposure to indoor or outdoor air pollution can have an immediate effect on a child, causing wheezing and shortness of breath in children without asthma and causing increased frequency and severity of asthma attacks in children who already have asthma. Air pollution can also cause bronchitis and pneumonia. The result is an increased number of school absences and hospitalizations.

Here are some of the effects of air pollution on asthma:

- The more severe the air pollution, the greater the number of asthma cases.
- Infants who are exposed to fine particulate air pollution have a greater chance of dying from sudden infant death syndrome (SIDS, or crib death).
- A woman exposed to air pollution during her pregnancy has a greater chance of having a premature delivery or a child with low birth weight.
- Children who are exposed to secondhand cigarette smoke have a higher rate of asthma than those not exposed to cigarette smoke.
- Inner city children who are exposed to high levels of air pollution from motor vehicles and industrial sources have higher rates of asthma and respiratory

disease hospitalizations than children in areas of low air pollution.

Reducing air pollution, even for a short period of time, reduces the number of hospitalizations of children due to asthma or respiratory disease. A few notable studies done in cities hosting Olympic games have definitively shown this.

In preparation for the 1996 Summer Olympics in Atlanta, the organizers worked with city officials to reduce air pollution by restricting motor vehicle traffic citywide during the games. This resulted in fewer hospital emergency room visits by children with asthma. (See Friedman et al., 2001, in Resources.)

Similarly, a study done during the 2008 Summer Olympics in Bejing, China, found that reducing outdoor air pollution, even for the short two-week period during the Olympics, resulted in fewer hospital emergency room visits by patients with asthma. (See Zheng et al., 2015, in Resources.)

Long-term reduction in air pollution can have great benefits for children's health. A study in Los Angeles showed that, between 2001 and 2008, as levels of air pollution came down, there were fewer pediatric hospitalizations for asthma than in previous years. When pollution rates were higher, there were more children hospitalized for asthma. (See Delamater et al., 2012, in Resources.)

The increasing rates of pollution in today's world are not good news for children with asthma. Added to that burden is the fact that some of the pollutants already released into the environment are persistent environmental pollutants that will remain in our bodies and in the bodies of our children and grandchildren for decades or even generations. Annual surveys done by the Centers for Disease Control and Prevention show that most people in the United States today carry measurable amounts of approximately 200 manufactured chemicals in their bodies. Some of the chemicals to which we are all widely exposed can tinker with our normal bodily processes.

Childhood Cancer

Rates of childhood cancer are increasing. Although new treatments for childhood cancer are giving hope to families and children for a long life, and death rates from childhood cancer are down, the number of new cancer cases per thousand children (the incidence rate) is on the rise. The single best way to protect children against cancer is to identify the causes of cancer and then to take action to prevent exposure to those causes.

Only 10% to 20% of cancers in children are considered to be genetic. The remaining 80% to 90% are due to environmental factors—chemical and physical factors in the environment called environmental carcinogens (carcinogens are cancer-causing substances or agents). Some environmental carcinogens, such as radiation, damage genes directly. Others become part of the cell and tinker with the switches that regulate genes, thereby confusing the normal developmental instructions given by natural body hormones. These epigenetic changes not only can damage the cell but also can affect the developing child, resulting in multiple types of health problems. But there are encouraging prospects here as well—we should be able to prevent cancers and other diseases caused by environmental sources by eliminating exposures to the environmental carcinogens once they are identified.

Now that the DNA of the human genome has been mapped, researchers have a powerful tool for identifying environmental carcinogens that are the causative agents in cancers. Research that focuses on gene–environment interactions can now be linked with information gained from population-based epidemiological studies. Researchers are working to analyze the mechanisms of the interaction between genes and the environment in order to understand how toxic chemicals in the environment cause childhood cancer, developmental delays, and reproductive dysfunctions, among others. This population-based genetic research will help define the link between childhood cancer and environmental toxins and will help identify additional toxic chemicals that may use the same mechanisms.

Most childhood cancer is diagnosed during the child's first five years of life, with a peak incidence during the first year. The most common childhood cancer is leukemia, followed by lymphomas and brain cancers.

There are known links between toxic chemicals and childhood cancers, but much more research is necessary to determine why childhood cancer is on the rise. Since many childhood cancers appear early in the child's life, research is focusing attention on prenatal exposures to cancer-causing agents as one piece in the puzzle of rising numbers of childhood cancer.

There are a number of known carcinogens (cancer-causing substances) that can increase the risk of cancer in children and adults. A partial list of carcinogens are discussed here in brief snapshots that incorporate information from the International agency for Research on Cancer, the National Cancer Institute, the Environmental Protection Agency, and the Centers for Disease Control and Prevention.

Aflatoxins are a group of toxic chemicals produced in warm, damp climates by various types of fungi and molds that grow on peanuts, corn, and other nuts. Aflatoxins can cause liver cancer in people who ingest contaminated food products. Cancer risk is greatest in people with liver damage or chronic infection with hepatitis B. Children can be exposed to aflatoxins in peanut butter made from peanuts contaminated with the fungus.

Air pollution is the aerosolized "toxic chemical soup" that we now all breathe. Outdoor air pollution includes breathable fine particulates of soot from vehicle exhaust and industrial smokestacks, as well toxic gases from fuel combustion—carbon dioxide, nitrogen oxides, carbon monoxides, and other chemical compounds. The reaction of these fine particulates and toxic gases with *ground-level ozone,* a respiratory irritant formed when ultraviolet light or electrical discharges react with oxygen, produces urban smog. Outdoor air pollution is a carcinogen.

Indoor air pollutants are also potentially toxic: carbon monoxide, radon, fumes from deodorizers, cleaners, household products, new building materials or furniture, household pest droppings, tobacco smoke, pollen, and mold.

A wide array of negative health effects—cancer, respiratory diseases, asthma, cardiovascular diseases, and premature birth have been linked to air pollution. Diesel exhaust is considered to be a proven lung carcinogen.

Anabolic steroids, particularly anabolic androgenic steroids used illegally by some athletes to enhance muscle bulk and improve performance, are carcinogenic. They have been shown to be a cause of liver cancer. Children and teens are at special risk because they may see steroids as a way to improve their athletic performance in competing for places on sports teams. In addition to the severe penalties for steroid use that are imposed by the governing bodies of organized sports, the health risks of steroid use are enormous. Steroids should never be used for any purpose having to do with athletics by persons of any age. The purported short-term gains are tiny compared with the damage steroids can cause.

Arsenic is a naturally occurring chemical element that can be found in air, water, and soil and that can cause cancers of the bladder, skin, lung, gastrointestinal system, liver, kidney, and blood. It occurs as a contaminant in water supplies, which can result in chronic exposure. It is also released into the environment by agricultural and smelting industries. Arsenic was used as a pesticide in the past and is still found in some manufactured products.

Children can be exposed to arsenic when they play near old wooden structures made of pressure-treated wood that was treated with chromated copper arsenate (CCA). Commonly used in earlier years for playground equipment and outdoor decks, CCA is an arsenic compound that can be ingested by children playing in the soil around the structures or from contaminated dust. Recent studies have shown that arsenic continues to leach from the treated wood for at least 7 to 10 years after installation.

Asbestos is the name given to a group of fibrous minerals that occur naturally in geologic formations around the world, but especially in Canada, Russia, Brazil, Western Australia, and South Africa. All types of asbestos are known carcinogens and must be carefully avoided. Asbestos fibers have been used extensively in the United States and elsewhere in shipbuilding and building construction since the early 20th century. Billions of tons of asbestos have been used in homes, public buildings, and schools in the United States and worldwide. Asbestos does not burn and is easily fabricated into insulation, fire-proofing, ceiling tiles, roof shingles, boiler coating, floor coatings, and spray-on wall and ceiling beam coverings.

As asbestos-containing tiles and insulation age and deteriorate, tiny, powdery fibers of asbestos are released into household air and house dust. When inhaled or ingested, these fibers can enter the body and remain dormant for decades. Up to 50 years later, they can cause lung cancer, gastrointestinal cancer, and malignant mesothelioma, a life-threatening cancerous tumor that is specific to asbestos.

Children are at risk of asbestos exposure from deteriorating ceiling coverings in older schools treated with asbestos and in multiple other buildings treated with asbestos products. Removal of asbestos should be done only by specially trained workers, ideally during school vations, since the dispersion of asbestos fibers during renovations or the demolishing of a building puts people exposed to the fibers at risk of cancer.

Aspartame is an artificial sweetener that has been widely used since the 1980s and is found today in thousands of products worldwide, notably in diet beverages. Previously it was considered safe, but large, long-term animal studies are now indicating that aspartame may be a potential cause of leukemia. Exposures to aspartame during pregnancy appear to especially hazardous and are associated in animal studies with increased rates of cancer in offspring.

Benzene is a thin, colorless, sweet-smelling solvent used in industry and manufacturing. Commercial products containing benzene include paint strippers, cleaners, adhesives, and glues. Exposure to benzene can cause leukemia, lymphoma, and other blood disorders.

Benzene was once a widely used solvent valued as a household spot remover and solvent for grease related to automotive or handyman projects in the home. However, the major risk to children today from benzene is through exposure to gasoline, which contains benzene. Children and teens can be exposed to benzene while pumping gasoline at a self-service station or when fueling small engines, such as lawnmowers. Benzene can also be absorbed into the body through the skin if fuel is splashed onto the skin.

Benzopyrene is a black, sooty, burnt substance that is formed when grilling food, burning toast, or roasting coffee and smoking tobacco. Car exhaust, wood fires, and forest fires can also contain benzopyrene. Benzopyrene has been linked to stomach and lung cancer.

Cadmium is a metallic element linked with bladder and possibly pancreatic cancer. A component of outdoor air pollution, cadmium is released into the environment from incinerators and zinc refineries. Commercial uses of cadmium include paint pigments, plastics, and batteries. Cadmium is also found in tobacco smoke.

DDT is an organochlorine pesticide that has been recently linked to breast cancer when exposure occurs early in life. Women who were exposed to DDT as young girls have a higher incidence of breast cancer in later life than other women. An elevated risk of breast cancer is also seen in women whose mothers who were exposed to DDT while they were pregnant with them. These findings demonstrate how toxic environmental exposures during windows of developmental vulnerability in early life influence risk of disease across the life span.

Diethylstilbesterol (DES) was a medication given in the 1960s and 70s to pregnant women who were in danger of having a miscarriage or spontaneous abortion. It is a known cause of vaginal cancer in young women who were exposed to it prenatally and it also causes some reproductive changes in males. There are some data indicating that the health effects of DES may be multigenerational.

Diesel exhaust contains dirtier and more toxic fumes than gasoline exhaust. Diesel exhaust is comprised of soot, carbon dioxide, carbon monoxide, several oxides of nitrogen and sulfur, formaldehyde, and benzopyrene. One of the most toxic components of diesel exhaust is 1,3-butadiene, a powerful carcinogen. Diesel exhaust has been classified as a known human carcinogen.

Dioxins are highly toxic, cancer-causing chemicals that are produced during the incineration of PVC plastics and other chlorine-containing compounds, such as PCBs. They are persistent organic pollutants (POPs) and have been found in milk, food, and even infant formula and breast milk. High-fat foods, such as meat, milk, and eggs, contain trace amounts of dioxins that are transferred to people who eat these foods. The Centers for Disease Control and Prevention annual survey lists dioxins as one of the 200 environmental chemicals found in the bodies of most Americans. (See also **TCDD**.)

Formaldehyde is a chemical widely used in household products, such as particleboard, pressed wood, plywood, glues, adhesives, paper products, insulation, and industrial resins. Perhaps it is best known as the chemical responsible for the "new furniture" or "new car" smell that is detected as newly purchased items release formaldehyde into the environment. Formaldehyde has been linked to leukemia and other cancers.

Lindane, also known as HCB (hexachlorobenzene), is an insecticide banned for agricultural use by the Environmental Protection Agency (EPA) in 1976 because it is a persistent organic pollutant. However, lindane is still available by medical prescription as a treatment for lice. It is a cause of liver cancer. Safer treatments for head lice now exist.

Nitrosamine is a toxic chemical produced in the body during the digestion of nitrate-containing preserved meats, such as hot dogs, luncheon meats, and sausages. This carcinogen is also found in tobacco smoke. Nitrosamines are classified as probable carcinogens linked to digestive system cancers.

PCBs (polychlorinated biphenyls) are highly chlorinated compounds formerly used in electrical insulation. They are highly persistent in the environment. They have been classified as carcinogens.

Perchloroethylene, also called PERC or tetrachloroethylene, is a solvent used in dry cleaning and metal degreasing. It is a probable carcinogen that may be linked to leukemia, bladder cancer, and lymphomas.

Pesticide exposure is linked various types of cancer, especially among farmworkers, their families, and people who live in agricultural areas. Several pesticides—glyphosate (Round-Up), malathion, and diazinon—have been classified as probable human carcinogens with links to lymphomas and other cancers. Tetrachlorvinphos and parathion are classified as possible carcinogens on the basis of data from animal studies.

Radiation has many forms, and each kind of radiation contains a specific amount and type of energy. The forms of radiation differ from one another in the ways they deliver energy to the human body and in the damage they produce.

Radiation causes injury to the body by transferring energy to the cells through which it passes. Different forms of radiation behave in very different ways, are found in different environmental settings, and can cause quite different types of injury. However, energy transfer is always the fundamental mechanism of radiation injury.

The transfer of energy that is produced by radiation is similar to other common energy transfers, such as the transfer of energy in a car crash or being hit by a baseball. When the moving object hits the body, it slows down by transferring its energy to the body's tissues and bones, causing cuts and abrasions or a broken bone. In a similar fashion, when a particle of radiation passes through the body, it collides with single atoms or molecules deep within the cells.

High doses of ionizing radiation, the type of radiation found in X-rays, radiation therapy, or atomic bombs, kill cells as it passes through the body. Deep burns, eye injury, and death from radiation sickness are some of the results. Destruction of bone marrow can occur. With the destruction of bone marrow, the body loses its ability to make new red and white blood cells; anemia and an impaired ability to fight off infection result. Destruction of the cell lining of the gastrointestinal tract is another feature of acute radiation sickness and this can cause death.

Lower-dose exposure to ionizing radiation causes subtle damage that may not appear for many years. At lower doses, radiation can alter and distort molecular structures within the cells of the human body. DNA, the fundamental human genetic material, is the most vulnerable target. When radiation strikes the nucleus of a cell, a change in DNA called a mutation occurs. Mutations caused by radiation can transform cells, leading to their becoming malignant and developing into widespread cancer.

In 1990 the National Academy of Sciences stated that there are no safe thresholds for exposure to ionizing radiation. Even the smallest doses are capable of causing mutations in DNA. In general, the higher the radiation dose, the more severe the effects on the human body, the greater the likelihood of mutation, and the greater likelihood of eventually developing cancer.

Exposure to ionizing radiation has been found to cause leukemia in children. Much of what we know about this link was learned years ago after massive radiation exposures in accidents or in time of war. Specific links between ionizing radiation and disease in children are the following:

- After the atomic bombings of Hiroshima and Nagasaki in World War II, there was an increase in leukemia in children that peaked seven years after the bombing. Later, incidence rates of certain solid tumors also increased.

- Studies in England have found that children of women who received abdominal X-rays during pregnancy have a greater chance of dying of leukemia in the first ten years of their lives than other children. The effect is seen at extremely low levels of radiation exposure. The finding led to a drastic deduction in the use of X-rays during pregnancy.
- When the Chernobyl nuclear power plant had a meltdown in the Ukraine in the 1980s, it released radiation in the form of radioactive iodine into the environment, contaminating towns and villages, people, farmlands, and animals. Children who were exposed to radiation from the Chernobyl meltdown showed elevated rates of thyroid cancer as teenagers.

Over the past decades, there has been a significant body of research on electromagnetic fields (EMFs), a form of non-ionizing radiation, to determine whether EMFs cause cancer. Although research results have been mixed, a recent study once again called attention to the potential risk of radiation from cell phones. It is prudent to limit children's exposure to EMFs and other forms of non-ionizing radiation.

Radon is a naturally occurring radioactive gas that is generated when naturally occurring uranium and other radioactive elements decay deep underground. Radon gas can seep up from underground deposits and be found in low levels in air, soil, and water in areas where geologic formations contain uranium. Radon seeps upward through cracks and gaps in the soil and can build up to toxic levels when it infiltrates indoor spaces, such as basements. Although engineering remedies exist to prevent its buildup in enclosed spaces, radon is second only to tobacco smoke as a cause for lung cancer in the United States.

Solvents are chemicals that are widely used in households and in industry to dissolve grease and other fatty substances.

Also called volatile organic compounds or VOCs, solvents vaporize readily and can enter the body through inhalation or through the skin. Even brief exposure to high levels of solvents can cause dizziness, nausea, hallucinations, and unconsciousness. Long-term exposure can cause damage to the nervous system and many solvents, including benzene, toluene, tricholoroethylene, and perchloroethylene, can cause cancers.

TCDD is an especially dangerous form of dioxin. Widespread exposures to TCDD occurred in a number of populations around the world. Studies have proven that TCDD is powerfully carcinogenic.

- During the Vietnam War in the 1970s, the herbicide Agent Orange was sprayed over large areas of Vietnam as a defoliant. Agent Orange was contaminated with TCDD which is a by-product of pesticide production. Subsequent large studies of the exposed Vietnamese population found elevated rates of lymphoma.
- In 1976, a chemical company manufacturing pesticides and herbicides in Seveso, Italy, exploded, spewing chemicals, including the dioxin contaminant TCDD, throughout the countryside. Thirty years later, a study of women who had been exposed prenatally to TCDD during the disaster showed an increased incidence of many different types of cancer, including lymphomas, leukemia, and other cancers.
- In the United States, a major episode of TCDD exposure occurred in Times Beach, Missouri, where chemical waste containing TCDD was sprayed on dirt roads during the summer months to hold down dust. The town became so contaminated that it had to be evacuated and destroyed.

Tobacco smoking still kills nearly 500,000 Americans annually—even though there are fewer tobacco smokers in American society and those who do smoke limit themselves to fewer cigarettes. Today's cigarettes are more lethal than previous cigarettes—their ventilated filters and chemical additives are contributing to an escalation in lung cancer rates.

Lung cancer, long the most common cancer in men, now surpasses breast cancer as the leading cancer in women. Smoking also dramatically increases the risk of stroke, heart disease, and chronic lung disease. The costs of tobacco to the American public are staggering, both in medical care costs and in years of life lost. Insurance companies long ago figured this out—life insurance has different prices for smokers and nonsmokers!

Parents need to know that about 90% of all cigarette smoking begins in childhood and adolescence. If a person is not already a smoker by his or her twenty-first birthday, it is highly unlikely he or she will ever become a smoker. It is essential that parents do everything they can to keep their children and teens from starting to smoke.

Smokeless tobacco, including snuff, is also a known cause of cancer and is strongly linked with cancer of the mouth and tongue (as well as to terrible bad breath). Furthermore, parents need to prevent children and teens from becoming addicted to e-cigarettes, too. E-cigarettes are far from innocuous. Smoking e-cigarettes, or vaping, is the tobacco industry's latest attempt at addicting a new generation of children and teens to nicotine. Vaping is an efficient drug-delivery system for aerosolized nicotine and other additives. It sends the toxic chemicals directly into the bodies of children and teens via their respiratory systems. The tobacco companies use tried-and-true marketing techniques—showing teen celebrities using the product, claiming that it is the "safer" way to smoke, and adding a wide variety of candy flavorings to provide "fun tastes" to hook children and teens on nicotine. Neither nicotine addiction nor tobacco smoking is safe or healthy for infants, children, teens, and adults.

One of the most important things that parents can do is to keep their children away from any form of tobacco.

Trichloroethylene (TCE) is a widespread industrial solvent that has contaminated thousands of groundwater systems across the United States. TCE is also a proven carcinogen.

It has been the suspected agent in multiple communitywide studies across the nation, in places where excess numbers of cancers or cancer clusters appeared. Although definitive studies of cancer clusters are complex, concerns about TCE contamination of water systems need to be resolved.

Ultraviolet light, a type of radiation, is a known cause of skin cancer. It is found in sunlight and also in the sunlamps used in tanning salons. Blistering sunburn in childhood and adolescence is linked with an increased incidence of skin cancer, especially malignant melanoma, in adult life. Tanning salons, which use artificial ultraviolet light for skin tanning, can cause skin cancer. The American Academy of Pediatrics strongly advises against any use of tanning salons for children under the age of 18 years.

Vinyl chloride is a chemical used in the production of polyvinyl chloride (PVC). It is a known carcinogen that causes liver cancer, brain cancer, and leukemia. It is an environmental air contaminant near PVC factories, a component of tobacco smoke, and a contaminant of water. If a water supply is contaminated with vinyl chloride, the chemical can be released as a vapor into the household when water is used for cooking or showering.

Although the above paragraphs are not an exhaustive list of the chemicals known to cause cancer, they do provide a starting point for investigating and eliminating the exposure of children to known cancer-causing chemicals.

Investigating the actual contribution of each of the possible chemicals and substances that may contribute to childhood cancer is a daunting challenge, but one that society should undertake sooner rather than later. The European community has shown that there are effective and feasible ways of prioritizing the list and making swift progress in getting suspect chemicals and known carcinogens out of the marketplace.

If future generations of children are to be protected against childhood cancers, research into the prevention of childhood cancer must be funded on at least an equal level with research into cancer treatment.

Neurodevelopmental Disorders

Chapter 3 discusses the early prenatal development of the infant and the intricacy of the clockwork precision needed during the nine months before birth for the infant to develop into a healthy newborn. The tiniest changes in this complex sequence of events—perhaps a momentary disruption of brain development caused by low-level exposure to lead, a pesticide or an endocrine-disrupting chemical—can interfere with normal development and cause serious damage.

So, preventing exposure during pregnancy and in early childhood to chemicals that can damage the brain is extremely important. For them to live a healthy and productive life, children need to have the best brain power possible.

Chemicals known to be linked neurodevelopmental disorders in children have already been mentioned as causing learning disabilities, sensory deficits, developmental delays, autism, and attention deficit/hyperactivity disorder. Exposures to these chemicals prenatally and in early childhood are the most dangerous. These environmental neurotoxins include:

Arsenic and **manganese.** Prenatal exposures to the metals arsenic and manganese are linked to neurodevelopmental impairment and reduced IQ in children. Manganese from industrial emissions or from some manganese-containing fungicides can harm a child's developing brain.

Bisphenol A, a synthetic chemical used to manufacture polycarbonate plastic, is linked to behavioral abnormalities and other problems described in the section "Reproductive Disorders and Endocrine Disruptors."

Brominated flame retardants. Prenatal exposure to brominated flame retardants has been linked to cognitive impairment, with lowered IQ and behavioral abnormalities.

Lead causes brain damage in children. The decades-long saga involving lead poisoning in children is a recurrent theme throughout this book. From the discovery in the early 20th century of lead poisoning in Australian children, to the removal of tetraethyl lead from gasoline in the 1970s, to the epidemic of lead poisoning in Flint, Michigan, in 2014, lead is now the best understood of all neurodevelopmental toxins. But the problem is still not solved. No level of lead is "safe."

The Centers for Disease Control and Prevention estimate that approximately 500,000 children in the United States still have elevated blood lead levels and are at risk of lead poisoning. These children, and generations of children before them, have or will suffer the effects of lead poisoning. Children of mothers who had lead poisoning in childhood are more likely to suffer neurodevelopmental disorders than children of unaffected mothers. Our jails and prisons hold a high proportion of adults who had lead poisoning as children, a situation described by Dr. Herbert Needleman, a pioneer in the study of lead poisoning. The neurobehavioral effects of lead poisoning are much better understood than are the results of exposure to other unknown chemicals in the environment. But lead-related damage will continue as long as there is lead in the paint and the plumbing of older houses, waiting to poison another child who moves in. Over 24 million housing units in the United States still contain lead; more than 4 million of these homes and apartments have children living in them.

Mercury is another well-studied toxic metal. Metallic mercury is toxic and vaporizes easily. It can cause neurological symptoms like those exhibited by the Mad Hatter in *Alice in Wonderland*, an apt characterization since hatmakers in the 19th century used metallic mercury to cure the felt used for men's top hats (such as the one worn by Abraham Lincoln).

Another form of mercury, methylmercury, is found in many contaminated lakes and streams due to the release of mercury-containing waste from factories and industries. Fish from these bodies of water cannot be eaten. The methylmercury accumulates up the food chain—larger fish eat contaminated smaller fish who have eaten contaminated algae, and so on, and levels of methylmercury can reach extremely high levels in the predator fish at the top of the food chain (Table 4-1). In the ocean, a similar course of events occurs—larger fish, such as swordfish, shark, king mackerel, and tilefish, may accumulate high levels of methylmercury and can pose a danger to the developing infant of a pregnant woman who eats the fish. Federal and state advisories warn of unsafe fish or suggest limits of the amount of fish that should be eaten by a pregnant woman. The most severe form of methylmercury poisoning was seen in Minimata, Japan, in 1956, where pregnant women who ate contaminated fish gave birth to severely neurologically damaged children. Several groups including the Natural Resources Defense Council and the Monterrey Bay Aquarium have published carefully researched lists showing which types of fish contain high levels of methyl mercury and which are safer to eat.

Polychlorinated biphenyls (PCBs). PCBs are a family of synthetic chemical compounds that contain chlorine. They are clear, oily, nonflammable liquids that resist heat and do not conduct electricity. They were widely used until the 1970s as liquid insulators in transformers, capacitors, and fluorescent light ballasts and are still found on older telephone poles and in the fluorescent fixtures in older schools throughout the country.

Table 4-1 Good Seafood Guide! (from the Environmental Working Group)

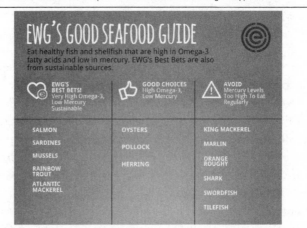

EWG'S GOOD SEAFOOD GUIDE

Eat healthy fish and shellfish that are high in Omega-3 fatty acids and low in mercury. EWG's Best Bets are also from sustainable sources.

EWG'S BEST BETS! Very High Omega-3, Low Mercury Sustainable	GOOD CHOICES High Omega-3, Low Mercury	AVOID Mercury Levels Too High To Eat Regularly
SALMON	OYSTERS	KING MACKEREL
SARDINES	POLLOCK	MARLIN
MUSSELS		ORANGE ROUGHY
RAINBOW TROUT	HERRING	
ATLANTIC MACKEREL		SHARK
		SWORDFISH
		TILEFISH

Over the years, large quantities of PCBs have been released into the environment from the factories that produced the PCBs, and from the breakdown of transformers, capacitors, and from ballasts, the units used to trigger fluorescent light-bulbs. The PCBs that have been released into the environment have washed into our harbors, lakes, and rivers and settled to the bottom, where they persist in the sediment. Although PCBs are no longer manufactured in the United States, they were used extensively for many years, and they continue to be important contaminants because they are persistent in the environment. PCBs do not break down, and they resist microbes that naturally destroy most chemical compounds, so they last in the environment for decades.

PCBs are soluble in fatty tissues, where they accumulate and move up the food chain. Like methylmercury, PCBs accumulate to high levels in certain species of fish. From the sediments at the bottom of the lakes and rivers they are taken up by worms, shellfish, catfish, and other bottom-feeding fish, including eels. When the bottom-dwellers are eaten by game fish, the PCBs accumulate to even higher levels in the fatty tissues of the predator species. Finally, when top predators such as eagles, ospreys, bears, or humans eat fish, they accumulate high levels of PCBs.

Human prenatal exposure to PCBs is principally the consequence of maternal consumption of contaminated fish before and during pregnancy. Prenatal exposure to PCBs is linked to reduction in children's intelligence.

Pesticides. Prenatal exposure to the organophosphate insecticide chlorpyrifos is associated with reduced head circumference at birth (an indicator of delayed brain development during pregnancy) and developmental delays. Prenatal chlorpyrifos exposures are also associated with cognitive impairments detectable at age 8 to 9 years, and with increased risk of autism spectrum disorder.

DDT exposure has been linked to increased risk of breast cancer in women who were exposed in early life. (See Cohn et al.,

2007, in Resources.) There is also a higher incidence of breast cancer in women whose mothers were exposed to DDT while they were pregnant with them. (See Cohn et al., 2016, in Resources.)

Phthalates. Baby boys prenatally exposed to phthalates, a widely used class of chemicals found in plastics, cosmetics, and many common household products, appear to be at increased risk of behavioral abnormalities that resemble attention deficit/hyperactivity disorder (ADHD) as well as other health problems described in the section "Reproductive Disorders and Endocrine Disruptors."

Perfluorinated chemicals, PFOA and **PFOS.** Prenatal exposures to the perfluorinated chemicals, PFOA and PFOS, have been linked to decreased birth weight and reduced head circumference in newborn infants. These chemicals are often used in nonstick cookware, weather-resistant fabric and clothing, and in other household applications.

Reproductive Disorders and Endocrine Disruptors

An endocrine disruptor is a chemical that mimics or blocks the action of the natural hormones in the human body. Natural hormones are powerful chemicals secreted in minute amounts by the body's endocrine glands—the pituitary, the thyroid, the pancreas, the adrenal glands, the ovaries, and the testes.

In the body, infinitesimal quantities of natural hormones control the whole range of growth, development, and reproduction, from prenatal development through adolescence, adulthood, and old age. Hormones are released into the circulation at precise times in development. They are extremely powerful chemicals. It is very worrisome that there are now scores of man-made, synthetic chemicals that can mimic and compete with natural hormones in the bodies of up to 90% of the world's population. In thinking about the possible effects of these endocrine disruptors, it is important to remember that the amount of a natural hormone needed to get the job done is minuscule by any standard. So the very presence in the body of low concentrations of synthetic chemicals that can mimic the actions of hormones is sufficient to cause concern and consternation.

There has been an explosion of interest in recent years in the developmental consequences of early-life exposures to chemicals that function as endocrine disruptors. Some specific examples of reproductive and endocrine disruptors are these:

Bisphenol A (BPA) is an endocrine disruptor used as an additive to polycarbonates and epoxy resins found in the plastic lining of food cans, in plastic tableware, in medical equipment, in toys, in food storage containers, in water supply pipes, and even in baby bottles. BPA can leach into the environment or into foods or liquids stored in containers with BPA in them. BPA is a persistent organic pollutant that can be found in nearly all residents of the United States.

Recent research shows that exposure to BPA prenatally and in early childhood is linked with aggression, hyperactivity, obesity, increased risk of cardiovascular disease, diabetes, and reproductive abnormalities that range from early puberty to sexual dysfunction and decreased levels of normal hormones.

Phthalates are endocrine-disrupting chemical compounds that are added to plastics to make them more flexible. Nearly all PVC products contain phthalates to make them more pliable, soft, and flexible. As the PVC ages, the product loses its plasticity, yellows, and becomes brittle—as many a consumer can attest when they look at the older plastic containers in their kitchen drawers. The yellowing is a visible marker of the leaching of the plastic's phthalates into the environment—and into your body and ours!

Other types of plastic and many other products contain types of phthalates that help them retain their color and scent. Phthalates are in widespread use in air fresheners, shampoos, perfumes, and cosmetics. The compounds don't stay in the products, and they release readily into the environment. People everywhere now have phthalates in their bodies—in measurable amounts.

Prenatal exposure to phthalates has been linked to shortening of the anogenital distance in baby boys, a finding indicative of decreased masculinization of the reproductive organs. This appears to be linked in adult life with lower sperm production and infertility. Neurodevelopmental changes are seen in later childhood, with feminized play in boys and attention deficit and aggressive behaviors in boys and girls. Overall, boys are more affected by phthalates than girls.

Childhood Obesity

For centuries, obesity was seen as a sign of health and wealth, indicating sufficient or even excessive food intake. The stereotype persists in many cultures around the world, with a chubby baby still being cherished as "the picture of health." Unfortunately, the reality is quite different.

Today, a global epidemic of childhood obesity is underway, with patterns of obesity and diabetes previously seen only in adults now developing in children worldwide. Obesity has more than tripled in American children since 1970. Type 2 diabetes, heart disease, cancers, and joint and mobility problems are the consequences of obesity and now plague the health of many children. If the current trend continues, today's generation of children may be the first generation of American children in over a century to have a shorter average life span than their parents.

The pathway to childhood obesity is complex. There are metabolic pathways relating obesity and diabetes that are being explored. The environment contributes to childhood obesity in several ways.

Today's "built environment" creates a much more sedentary lifestyle for our children than for the children of previous generations. Urban housing with unsafe outdoor playgrounds, parks, and walking areas breeds a generation of latchkey children who return from school to the safety of indoors, where their playtime consists of watching television, playing computer games, and snacking on high-calorie commercial snacks. Sprawling suburban communities without sidewalks and with no town or village centers within walking distance require auto-mobiles to access the necessities of life: grocery stores, shopping malls, schools, playgrounds, distant parks. The lack of inter-esting, natural outdoor play spaces like vacant lots, woodland paths, or waterfronts where a child has the freedom to explore the world with other children leads to an increase in attention deficit disorder, anxiety, and depression—and obesity.

But research is also beginning to shed light on some other factors that may contribute to obesity. Some early-life expo-sures to environmental chemicals that can act as "obesogens" are now linked with a tendency toward both childhood and adult obesity. Obesity has been linked also with maternal smok-ing during pregnancy, exposures to PCBs and phthalates—both ever-present in our environment and in the bodies of almost all of us—and to organochlorine pesticides, such as DDT, found in most people around the world today since they persist in the food supply (despite having been banned in the United States over 20 years ago). Another organochlorine pesticide, lindane (or HCB, hexachlorobenzene), is still very present in our envi-ronment. Most recently, air pollution—which carries a load of multiple toxic chemicals—has been linked with obesity.

What are the most pressing questions about the links between environmental chemicals in use in commercial products today and childhood disease?

Here are some of the specific questions that are still un-answered:

Asthma and other respiratory diseases
- Why have asthma rates continued to rise in places where air pollution is coming under control?
- What are the still undiscovered causes of childhood asthma?
- What air pollution control strategies will be most effec-tive in reducing childhood asthma?

Childhood Cancer

- Why has the incidence of childhood cancer continued to rise more or less steadily over the past 40 years? None of the currently identified risk factors accounts for more than a fraction of this increase.
- What are the still undiscovered toxic risk factors for childhood cancer?

Neurodevelopmental Disorders

- What toxic chemicals contribute to the causation of autism?
- What toxic chemicals contribute to the causation of ADHD?
- What are the still undiscovered toxic chemical risk factors for neurodevelopmental disorders in children?

Obesity and Diabetes

- What is the contribution of chemical obesogens to rising rates of childhood obesity and diabetes?
- What is the contribution of air pollution to obesity?

Reproductive Problems

- Why are rates of hypospadias and testicular cancer rising?
- Why are sperm counts falling?

It is not easy to predict the extent to which these questions may be linked to environmental exposures, but the answers are important.

What are the next frontiers of research in understanding how environmental exposures can cause disease in children?

- **Gene–environment interactions.** Advances in biotechnology have enabled researchers to look at the actual interactions between environmental agents and genes. It

is useful to remember that environmental interactions can be specific to an individual's genetic makeup. Not everyone exposed to a toxic chemical develops the same injury.
- Gene–environment interactions can be divided into two types. The first are those that involve actual physical damage (a mutation) in the gene, such as the changes that are caused by ionizing radiation and benzene. The second type are changes caused by the agents that get into the cells (epigenetic agents) and play with the switches that turn various genes "on" and "off"—sometimes getting stuck in the "on" position.

Maternal smoking may prove to be an epigenetic agent. There is a known link between childhood obesity and maternal smoking during pregnancy, but the exact mechanism is not yet known. We do know that maternal smoking constricts the blood flow from the mother to the placenta, thus reducing the supply of oxygen and nutrition available to the developing child. It is also known that when the developing child is not getting enough nutrition from a mother, nature can turn on a gene switch or a combination of switches that put the developing baby into caloric overdrive to survive the ordeal. If the switch gets stuck in the "on" position after birth, it could cause the child to continue to pile up available calories into fat, leading to obesity, hypertension, cardiac problems, and diabetes as the child grows up. By reducing the availability of nutrition to the developing child, maternal smoking very likely triggers nature's survival mechanism leading to obesity, hypertension, cardiac problems, and diabetes in later years.

- **Epigenetic changes that can have devastating effects on the body.** Phthalates, bisphenol A, and other endocrine disrupting chemicals can tinker with gene switches that affect the developing baby's reproductive system. Confused signaling may cause sexual identity problems in childhood, attention deficits, aggressive behaviors, low sperm counts in adult males, infertility, early puberty, and other already identified problems with the reproductive system.

Is there evidence that harmful environmental exposures in early life cause disease in adult life?

Diseases now suspected to be influenced in part by early environmental exposures include diabetes, cardiovascular disease, dementia, Parkinson disease, and cancer. The *developmental origins of adult disease theory* represents an extension of landmark observations made by Professor David Barker and his colleagues at the University of Southampton, United Kingdom, who found that the prenatal nutritional environment can influence health throughout the life span. (See Barker, JD in Resources.)

Increasing incidence rates of certain cancers and also of Parkinson disease and Alzheimer disease are of great concern. These trends are too rapid to be of genetic origin. The findings raise the possibility that environmental exposures—including exposures in fetal and early postnatal life—may be contributing to noncommunicable diseases in adult life, even into extreme old age.

A possible mechanism connecting early exposures with late effects is that early exposures may initiate cascades of changes within cells that can lead ultimately to malignancy or that can reduce the numbers of neurons in critical areas of the brain to levels below those needed to maintain function in the face of advancing age. Some of the changes may be mediated by epigenetic modulation of gene expression by toxic chemicals or other environmental exposures.

What are the economic costs of childhood diseases caused by toxic chemicals in the environment?

Diseases in children caused by toxic chemicals in the environment carry very great economic costs. Development of information on the costs of disease is important in the formulation of health policy and for convincing policymakers, who must make hard choices among many competing demands, that childhood diseases of toxic environmental origin should be a high priority.

A recent analysis of the medical and societal costs associated with four categories of illness of environmental origin in American children—lead poisoning, asthma, cancer, and neurobehavioral disorders—found the costs to amount to $76.6 billion annually.

The principal contributor to the costs is the lifelong reduction in intelligence that results from exposures in early life to neurotoxic chemicals that erode intelligence, such as lead, methylmercury, and PCBs. Widespread loss of intelligence imposes great burdens on society for services, such as vocational training and special education, and leads to lifelong reduction in economic productivity.

Conversely, what are the economic benefits of preventing disease in children caused by toxic chemicals in the environment?

On the positive side, prevention of environmental disease can yield great economic benefit. Grosse et al. have estimated that the increases in children's intelligence and thus in lifetime economic productivity that resulted from the removal of lead from gasoline have produced an economic benefit of between $110 and $319 billion in each US birth cohort born since the 1980s through the increased intelligence, creativity and economic production of generations of children who have grown up with only low-level exposures to lead. The cleaning of America's air that followed passage of the Clean Air Act amendments of 1990 is estimated to have yielded cost savings of $2 trillion, mainly in reduced healthcare costs and increased economic productivity—an economic befit of about $30 for every dollar invested in pollution control.

5

LEAD IN THE HOME

Lead is a toxic metal. It can permanently damage a child's brain, heart, and kidneys. At high levels, lead poisoning can cause seizures, coma, and even death.

But even small amounts of lead can harm children. The brain is especially sensitive. Studies have shown that children with even low levels of lead in their blood have more difficulty learning and that they lose an average of 2 to 4 points in their IQ for every 10-microgram increase of their blood lead levels. It is now known that there is no safe level of lead in the blood. Low levels of lead in the blood have also been linked to short attention span and aggressive behavior. Researchers have shown that young men under age 18 jailed for juvenile delinquency have higher levels of lead in their bodies than other young men from the same neighborhood without a criminal record.

There have been historic gains in the battle to eliminate childhood lead poisoning, but there are still approximately 500,000 children in the United States with elevated levels of lead in their blood, with more found every day.

And outbreaks of lead poisoning still occur. The most recent was in Flint, Michigan.

The 2014 tragedy in Flint, in which a city manager made a short-sighted and budget-driven decision to switch the source of the city's drinking water supply from the clean water of the

Great Lakes and Detroit River to the polluted water of the Flint River, turned a painful spotlight on both the perils of lead exposure and the continuing burdens of lead poisoning in poor and minority communities. The Flint River, rendered highly acidic by decades of industrial dumping, dissolved lead from ancient lead pipes in the city's aging infrastructure, thereby sharply increasing the concentrations of lead in the public's drinking water. Families were not aware that lead levels in their water had increased, and the water company denied the existence of any problem. As a result, families in Flint continued to use tainted water for many months, and between 6,000 and 12,000 children were exposed to high levels of lead in their water and were placed at increased risk of lead poisoning and permanent damage to their brains and nervous systems before the problem was discovered.

The lead exposure in Flint was an avoidable and unnecessary epidemic that put thousands of children at great risk. But it was not an isolated episode: lead poisoning in America is still alive and well. As long as there is lead paint in old buildings, there are lead pipes in our drinking water system, and there is lead in the soil, the effects of lead poisoning will continue to be seen.

The obvious remedy for this silent epidemic is individual and community vigilance in recognizing and removing lead wherever it is found. What follows is a practical guide to spotting and preventing lead poisoning.

How do I know if my home has lead in it?

Lead paint and the dust that forms when lead paint chips and erodes are the most common causes of lead poisoning. Luckily, because lead paint chips and peels as it ages, it often—but not always—makes its presence known. Check for peeling and chipping paint inside and outside your house.

Older homes are the most likely to contain lead paint because the federal government didn't ban residential uses of lead-based paint in the United States until 1978. Lead paint in houses deteriorates over time; it creates lead dust and chips that fall on the floor and collect in window wells and on windowsills, floor moldings, and other flat places (Figure 5-1). Young children, especially infants and children less than 6 years old, are at greatest health risk from lead paint and dust.

Lead paint gets into the bodies of children in a variety of ways. Kids can ingest the lead-tainted dust after putting toys contaminated by lead dust in their mouths, or by putting their fingers in their mouths after crawling around the floor. Infants and toddlers put everything in their mouths; it's their way of exploring the world. When toddlers are tall enough to stand up and look out the window, the windowsill might double as a teething ring. If there is lead paint or lead in the dust on the windowsill, it is a ready source of lead poisoning.

So normal childhood behaviors can result in lead poisoning if there is lead in the paint in your house. Compounding this problem is the fact that lead paint chips taste sweet. Some children can actually develop a craving for lead paint chips—this is called *pica*. Kids with pica will seek, find, and eat tiny

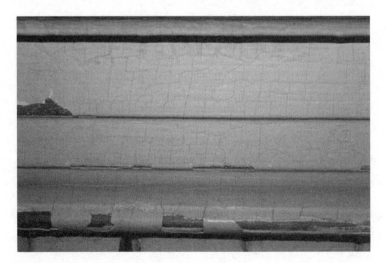

Figure 5-1 Typical cracking in old lead paint

chips of lead paint that are around. Kids with pica like the taste of lead paint so much that they become quite persistent in finding tiny chips that might escape adult notice.

So the best way to protect an infant and toddler from lead paint poisoning is to make sure that lead isn't in your home at all - ideally before you move in.

Where is lead typically found in a home?

Window wells. The window well is the part of the window that is exposed at the bottom when you open the window. So open the window and take a peek. Is the window well painted? If so, does the paint look cracked or crazed, like the skin of an alligator? Are there any chips of paint visible? Do there seem to be many layers of paint in the well? If so, this area may contain lead paint.

Window and door frames. Is there flaking, peeling, or chipping paint where friction occurs? Is there visible chipping, flaking, cracking, or crazing anywhere on the frames? Is there paint dust on the floor or wall molding?

Plaster walls. Pay particular attention to areas under the windows and in places where leaks or moisture may have caused some damage to the surface of the paint. Are chips, flakes, or plaster or paint dust apparent?

Stairs, banisters, wainscoting, old cast-iron radiators, and chair rails. Again, look for signs of flaking, peeling, and chipping paint. Also check out other painted wooden surfaces in your house that are subject to wear and tear. Opening and closing of doors, windows, closets, cabinets, and other moveable painted fixtures cause friction that wears the lead paint down into dust, which then disperses through the house. Do you see any worn areas of paint?

The outside of your house. Lead paint may also have been used on the trim or siding of the house, if your house was built before 1978. Again, look for signs of flaking, peeling, and chipping paint. Is the paint trim around windows and doors chipping or crazed? Are there multiple, lumpy layers of paint on trim? Check the garage and garden storage areas also, as well as fences and porch railings. Take a good look at the sandbox or play area—is it so close to the house that it might be contaminated by paint chips or paint dust from the house trim? (A word of caution here—just because you do not see evidence of lead paint, it does not mean that lead paint is not present in your home. If your home was built before 1978, the safer course is to have the house inspected top to bottom for lead by a certified professional.)

What do I do if I find evidence of lead paint in my home?

If you find peeling, chipping, or crazed paint in your house or your house was built before 1978, it's important to first confirm that the paint is lead. If you don't own your own home or apartment, let your landlord know if you've seen signs of peeling or chipping paint that might indicate lead paint and ask him or her for evidence that the home or apartment has been tested for lead paint. If it hasn't been tested, ask to have it done.

What actions you take for your home and your child(ren) will be partly defined by where you live. The Environmental Protection Agency (EPA) offers a resource (www.epa.gov/lead) on what interventions are available to you as an apartment dweller or homeowner to prevent lead poisoning. A city or state health department may also have a childhood lead poisoning prevention program that might have information for you—call them. A list of the ten regional EPA offices across the United States and information about which states each office serves are provided in the Resources section of this book.

If you own your house or apartment, you'll want to find an EPA-certified or state-certified lead inspector who has been trained in lead paint assessment and abatement. (The EPA requires that workers who perform lead paint assessment and lead paint abatement projects in housing built before 1978 be certified by EPA or by an EPA-authorized state and that they follow specific lead-safe work practices.) If you live in Alabama, Delaware, Georgia, Iowa, Kansas, Massachusetts, Mississippi, North Carolina, Oklahoma, Oregon, Rhode Island, Utah, Washington, Wisconsin, or the tribal territory of Bois Forte Band, your state is one of the EPA-authorized states that run their own certification programs; the EPA website will direct you to a site that contains specific information for your own state. The bottom line here is to make sure you use a contractor who has passed the EPA-certified or state-certified courses and training guidelines that ensure that he or she is qualified to do the job. Ask to see the documentation of his certification.

Make sure your pediatrician knows the details of your housing situation—that your home or apartment has or has not been tested for lead paint, how old your house is, and what you know about lead paint hazards. Ask your child's pediatrician about how often your child should be tested for lead and at what ages. Being proactively involved in protecting your child from lead paint is the best way to prevent lead poisoning.

What is the correct way to remove lead paint?

If an EPA-certified lead inspector determines that you have lead in your home, ask for a risk assessment and options for handling the problem. These reports, from EPA-certified risk assessment specialists, offer effective analysis of what needs to be done to protect your children from lead poisoning. This report, brought to an EPA-certified lead abatement contractor, will offer a roadmap to effective lead abatement.

Some additional things to keep in mind:

- Don't ever try to remove lead paint by yourself.
- Lead paint should never be sanded or removed with a heat gun. Both of these techniques can create highly hazardous lead dust or lead vapor that can spread through

the house and cause lead poisoning in you and your children.

Can children or pregnant women stay in a home during lead abatement?

No. Children and pregnant women must live with relatives or friends while the EPA- certified lead abatement specialists are working. They shouldn't return or even visit until all the debris and dust have been thoroughly cleaned up and the house is certified as safe from lead hazards. Because a child's brain and nervous system are still developing, direct exposure to lead dust is a risk for lead poisoning. And if a pregnant woman experiences a severe case of lead poisoning, she may have a miscarriage, stillbirth, premature delivery, or premature rupture of her membranes. At lower levels of lead poisoning, the baby's developing brain and nervous system can be irreversibly damaged.

How does lead get into drinking water?

Some older communities have lead pipes delivering water from the municipal water treatment plants to homes. Over the years, the pipes become coated on the inside with a biofilm, a layer of organic material that acts as a protective coating to keep the lead from coming in direct contact with the water. In places where the municipal water is acidic, however, the acidity eats away at the biofilm, causing the lead to dissolve from the pipes into the water. This is what happened in Flint, Michigan, in 2014.

Most lead in drinking water, though, comes from pipes and plumbing within schools, homes and apartment buildings. In the early and mid 1900s, lead pipes were commonly used in household plumbing. So if you have an old house and the plumbing system has never been updated, you might still have lead pipes conducting water from the city water mains into your faucets.

Lead pipes are generally a dull gray color and the metal is somewhat soft. Other materials used for household plumbing include cast iron and copper. Cast-iron pipes are usually black and hard. Copper piping is the traditional copper color. (But note: even if you have copper piping, you might still have lead in your water because there may have been lead in the solder used to join the pipes together. Lead solder has been banned only since 1986.)

If you have lead or copper pipes in your house, you'll want to know for certain if they're leaching lead into your water. If you are served by municipal water, you should receive notification from your city's water supplier if you have lead in your water. In 1991 the Environmental Protection Agency put into effect its Lead and Copper Rule, which requires water suppliers to notify their customers if lead or copper levels in their water exceed standards set by the federal government. In addition, all water companies are required to send out an annual report on contaminants to their customers. Another resource is the Environmental Working Group's National Tap Water database released in 2017, available at ewg.org/consumer guides. It provides information on chemical contaminants in drinking for water systems across the United States.

If you have well water, you should have your water tested for lead content by a certified laboratory. There have been many instances of well water being contaminated by toxic chemicals from factories, gasoline stations and hazardous waste sites, and because chemicals can travel long distances through aquifers, the source may be far away from the contaminated well. Contact your local or state health department for a list of certified laboratories near you or visit www.epa/lead to get information on certified lead testing labs.

Having lead in your water doesn't necessarily mean you need to replace the plumbing in your home. In most cases, the easiest way to eliminate any lead in your drinking water or cooking water before using it for drinking or cooking is to run the cold water for 30 seconds or so to flush out the line carrying the water after it has sat in the pipes for hours at a time—such as after work or school and the first thing in the morning. Because water from a municipal water supplier is generally lead-free when it leaves the water treatment plant, running the water before using it lets you access lead-free water that hasn't been sitting in your household plumbing overnight or for hours at a time, which allows time for lead to leach from your household pipes or lead-based pipe solder. And *always* use cold water to drink, cook, and make baby formula—hot water can leach more lead from the household plumbing. (If you're on a well, you should still run the water for 30 seconds after its been sitting for a while to be safe.)

Can lead exposure be tested for medically?
Should I have my child tested for lead?

Yes. The best way to test for lead in the human body is by a blood lead test.

The only way to be sure a child doesn't have lead poisoning is to have her pediatrician test her blood for lead, using the guidelines from CDC currently in place. The blood lead test is especially important for children between the ages of 1 and 3 if they live in homes built before 1978 because children in this age group living in older homes are at the highest risk for lead poisoning.

It's good practice for children to have a blood lead test done at 1 year of age and again at 18 months to 2 years of age. The test involves taking only a few drops of blood from a child's fingertip. Most pediatricians will be happy to do the test.

Lead poisoning is a very old problem, but what is new is our ability today to test for lead exposure and lead poisoning using sophisticated analyses. The results of these analyses are alarming.

Over the course of the past few decades, the Centers for Disease Control and Prevention (CDC) have repeatedly lowered the acceptable blood lead levels in children. These repeated reductions reflect the fact that we now know more than we did 5 or 10 years ago, and much more than 25 years ago, about the toxicity of lead at low levels. Blood lead levels that were once considered safe for children are now known to be dangerous. Medical researchers now understand that there is no safe level of lead in blood. The World Health Organization has echoed this conclusion.

Two generations ago, when leaded gasoline was in general use, the average blood lead level for Americans of all ages was between 18 and 20 µg/dL and some children had blood levels over 40 µg/dL.

A generation ago, after the removal of lead from gasoline, the average blood lead level of most people in the United States, including most children between 1 and 5 years old, was close to 20 µg/dL. Today, the average blood lead level in American children is below 2 µg/dL, a decrease of more than 90%.

Unfortunately, there are still about 500,000 children in the United States with elevated blood lead levels. These children are at risk of lead poisoning from lead in their homes. Most of them have no symptoms.

I have lead in my home. What do I do in the interim between discovery and abatement?

The safest solution is to temporarily relocate until the paint problem is abated. Any other option comes with risks.

If it is necessary to stay in the home for a brief time before abatement, make every effort to minimize the risk to your child. Frequent wet mopping will help to keep the dust down while you make arrangements for the certified lead paint assessment and risk reduction specialist to make your house safe. Mop at least weekly with a damp mop and mild detergent solution from the floor up the walls to the height of your child plus one foot. Many grocery stores and home centers carry nontoxic green soaps you can dilute with water to make a mild cleaning solution. Wet mopping will help get rid of some dust before it gets into your child. Unless you have a vacuum with a good

HEPA filter, wet mopping is safer than stirring up the dust with a conventional vacuum cleaner.

Remember that wet mopping is not a permanent way to fix the problem—it's like putting on a bandage or a tourniquet on a cut until you get to the emergency department. It's prudent to do everything you can while you make arrangements for a more proper abatement—but mopping up the dust does NOT solve the problem. The methods discussed here are only a *temporary* way to try to minimize the damage. The solution to the problem is the proper removal of lead as soon as feasible.

Along with wet mopping floors, use paper towels dampened with a cleaning solution to wipe down window wells, baseboards, floor and door moldings, wall trims, and other flat places. Seeing things from your child's point of view will also help you figure out which nooks and crannies to clean. Sit on the floor and move around the room, removing dust from every place your child can reach. Put the used paper towels in a secure trash container so they don't dry out and redistribute the lead dust around the house.

In addition, regularly wash your child's toys and pacifiers. Wash your child's hands frequently as well, especially before he sits down for a meal or snack.

These measures are not the solution to the problem, but they can't hurt. The best thing you can do in the interim between finding the problem and having it solved is to relocate to a safer place. This is by far the best option if you are pregnant or have young children.

Do children's toys contain lead?

In recent decades, lead has been trickling into the United States via toys manufactured in China and other less-regulated countries. Recalls or product warnings due to lead content have included:

- Crayons made in China
- China tea sets for doll houses

- Painted toys imported from Mexico and China
- Lead figurines used in adventure games for children and teens

What other imported items contain lead?

Pottery made in the United States is required to pass inspections that ensure it is lead-free; but this is not always the case in other countries, and imported pottery has been known to contain lead. Additionally, when pottery's glazing is imperfect, lead from the paint under the glaze can come in contact with your food.

The greatest danger with improperly glazed pottery is using it to store acidic liquid—for example, orange juice stored in a pottery pitcher. The acid in the orange juice can dissolve the lead, making it more readily and heavily consumed later. In general, don't use pottery that is not made in the United States for storing any acidic liquid.

The US Food and Drug Administration (FDA) warns that consumers should pay particular attention to ceramic ware or pottery that is:

- Handmade, with a crude appearance or irregular shape
- Antique
- Damaged or excessively worn
- Purchased from flea markets or street vendors or if you are unable to determine whether the pottery is from a reliable manufacturer
- Brightly decorated in orange, red, or yellow glaze, as lead is often used with these color pigments to increase their intensity.

The CDC and the FDA have also issued warnings that lead has been found in some imported consumer products, such as:

Imported candles. Some candles manufactured in poorly regulated countries include lead in their wicks. A leaded wick can produce lead fumes as it is burned, causing a serious hazard if the fumes are inhaled. Although the Consumer Product Safety Commission voted to ban candles like these, they still appear in some settings, and you should still make sure that any candles you buy are certified lead-free.

Imported candies and spices. Lead has been found in some imported candies and spices from Mexico and elsewhere, as well as chili powder and tamarind. Lead gets into these products when the drying, storing, and grinding of the ingredients are done improperly. Lead has also been found in the wrappers of some imported candies. The ink of the plastic or paper wrappers may contain lead that leaches into the candy.

Traditional health remedies and cosmetics. Some health remedies used traditionally in other countries, such as *azarcon* and *greta*—which are used for gastrointestinal upsets—contain lead and should not be used. Lead and other toxic metals are also found in some Ayurvedic medicines from South Asia.

A cosmetic called *kohl* (also called *kajal, al-Kahal, surma, tiro, tozali,* and *kwalli*) from parts of Africa, the Middle East, Pakistan, and India also contains lead and should not be used. There have also been reports of lead in other imported cosmetics, such as lipstick. The United States Food and Drug website, www.fda.gov, is a good resource for more information on this topic.

6

ALLERGENS AND RESPIRATORY IRRITANTS AT HOME

Children are more susceptible to air pollutants than adults. Children live closer to the ground, breathe far more air pound per pound of body weight, have lungs that are still developing, and have body organs that are not able to fend off pollutants. A child's vulnerability to air pollutants reveals itself in attacks of asthma, allergies, or both.

The allergy or bodily response to the allergen may be as mild as itchy eyes, a runny nose, and sneezing, or as severe as asthma. Some allergies, such as peanut allergy, can even be life-threatening. Common allergens include plant pollens, dust mites, molds, and some foods. This chapter discusses allergens that cause respiratory distress.

Asthma has both a genetic and an environmental component. From a genetic standpoint, children whose mothers or fathers had asthma as children are more likely to have asthma than children whose parents had no history of asthma. The environmental component is equally compelling. Children whose mothers or fathers smoked during pregnancy or during the first years of the child's life are much more likely to have asthma than children whose parents did not smoke.

Research also shows that repeated exposures to substances in the environment that produce allergic reactions can cause a child's airway to become inflamed and react with greater and greater severity each time the child is exposed to the allergen.

Some of the most potent allergens associated with asthma attacks in children are tobacco smoke, dust mites, cockroaches, and furry animals.

The environmental components of asthma and allergies are things that can be addressed and in some cases eliminated. Some changes are easy to make, while others may alter a family's lifestyle in a significant way. The recommendations here are guidelines, not hard and fast rules to be followed without careful thought.

Is the air in my home polluted?

Before you say no to this question, consider that in most areas, indoor air has more pollutants than outdoor air. If you have any of these inside your home, you may have air pollution:

Rugs and carpets	Furniture
Curtains	Dog and cat hair
Cleaning products	Cockroach droppings
Nail polish remover	Secondhand cigarette smoke
Hair spray	Furnaces
Shoe polish	Gas stoves
Potpourri	Wood-burning stoves and fireplaces
Air fresheners	

In other words, almost all homes have some sources of indoor air pollution. The simplest way to prevent the pollutants from building up is to air out your house or apartment thoroughly once a week.

To air out your house, it's best to choose a bright, clear day with a light wind. Open your windows and let the air blow through your house. In an apartment without cross-ventilation, you could strategically place a window fan in one window, to blow the outdoor air in, and another window fan in a more distant window, to draw the air out. Try to create a good draft to change the air in the room.

On cold winter days, you might even consider turning off your heat for an hour or two and airing out the house. To conserve household heat, do this during the mildest day of the week. Choose a sunny day, open your window shades at the same time on the sunny side and bask in the free solar heat it brings into your house.

During hot summer days, choose a relatively cooler day to turn off air conditioning. Close the curtains on the sunny side of the house and open up the house on the shady side to let the cool air clear out the pollution.

Of course, sometimes the outdoor air quality won't be very good. Pollen in the air, for example, can cause allergies. The weather report on your local news channel or the national Weather Channel is often a good source of information on the pollen count in your area. If your child is allergic to pollen, you may have to adjust your house-airing accordingly.

Ozone levels and particulate air pollution are two other sources of air pollution to consider before opening up your house. Ozone is a respiratory irritant that is formed when sunlight reacts with automobile exhaust fumes and industrial pollution in the atmosphere. In some parts of the country, "ozone alerts" or "air particulate" alerts are issued. They are common during the hot, humid days of summer. Listen for the alerts and don't air out your house when ozone or fine particulate matter levels are high.

What are the effects of smoking indoors on air quality?

Children who live in households with smokers are at a much greater risk than other children of developing asthma and other respiratory diseases. Children have a lifetime ahead of them for the harmful products contained in tobacco smoke to wreak havoc on their bodies.

Tobacco smoke isn't the only smoke in a house that can cause problems, however. Here are other common sources of smoke that can be devastating to a child's health:

Wood-burning stoves and fireplaces are a joy to watch on a cold night, but can give off all kinds of toxic materials, including fine particulate air pollution, benzopyrene (black soot), benzene, formaldehyde, and carbon monoxide. Children who are exposed to wood smoke are more likely than other children to have chronic cough, wheezing, and asthma attacks. These children may also be at greater risk for lung cancer, because the tars and tiny particles produced in wood smoke are similar to those produced in tobacco smoke.

Wood-burning stoves and fireplaces can be used without endangering the health of a child. First, make sure the wood-burning stove or fireplace has an adequate draft. The smoke should go up the chimney, not into the room. Second, if you have a wood-burning stove, have the catalytic converter and chimney checked and cleaned at least once a year to make sure they are working as efficiently as possible and to reduce the risk of fire. You also might want to visit the Environmental Protection Agency's website at www.epa.gov/burnwise for regulatory information on wood-burning stoves and ideas on more efficient models.

Fumes from stoves and furnaces can also contain carbon monoxide. This odorless, colorless gas cannot be detected before it reaches lethal levels, which is why it's extremely dangerous. Your best defense against potential problems with carbon monoxide fumes from gas stoves, wood stoves, furnaces, and water heaters is to have them checked annually for proper combustion and venting. Old chimneys can develop leaks, and chimney flues can become clogged, too, allowing life-threatening carbon monoxide to seep into your house. So it's also important to have your chimney cleaned and checked annually. And it's well worth it to invest in one or more carbon monoxide detectors with a digital readout and an audio alarm that will alert you to dangerous levels of the gas. A digital readout enables you to detect the actual level of carbon monoxide in the room and will help you determine whether you have a severely malfunctioning unit or one that is producing borderline elevations. You might also want to check *Consumer Reports* for information about specific models and their performances.

Gas stoves produce nitrogen dioxide fumes and other respiratory irritants. Some stoves have a constantly burning gas pilot light. These are particularly troublesome since they produce irritants day and night. If you have a gas stove with a pilot light, frequently ventilate your house to help reduce irritants. And the next time you buy a gas stove, you may wish to choose one without a pilot light. Instead of a pilot light, a stove can have an electronic ignition system that produces a spark when you turn on the burner—the spark then ignites the gas burner.

Oil-burning furnaces produce fumes that can be toxic if you don't have adequate ventilation in your home. Spilled or leaking fuel oil can introduce toxic chemicals into the air; it can also find its way into well water if there are wells in the vicinity of the spill. Scrupulous maintenance of your oil burner, annual checkups on efficiency and ventilation, and regular cleanings for the chimney and filters are the best way to prevent problems with your oil furnace.

Gasoline and kerosene home heaters (space heaters) are very dangerous from a fire safety standpoint and also produce toxic substances—including soot, which can cause cancer, and carbon monoxide, which can cause death by asphyxiation. Gasoline and kerosene heaters can accidentally tip over, spilling fuel and causing terrible burns and house fires. The best defense is to avoid using these heaters. If you currently have a gasoline or kerosene heater, replace it with an electric heater that doesn't get hot to the touch.

Do everyday household products pollute the air in a home?

They can, yes. The following is a discussion of household products that contain respiratory irritants and toxic chemicals, along with hints on how you can minimize the dangers from them.

Drain cleaners. Drain cleaners that contain lye (sodium hydroxide) are some of the deadliest home products on the market. Your best bet when it comes to drain cleaners is to avoid using them. The lye in most drain cleaners can cause severe burns and can cause life-threatening internal burns if a child drinks it. When the product is used in a clogged drain, it can produce toxic fumes that rise out of the drain. Instead, try a nontoxic method of fixing the problem. Pour 1 cup of baking soda and 1 cup of vinegar down the drain. Follow them with boiling water to help break the clog. If your sink is draining slowly, you could also take apart the U-shaped trap beneath the sink and remove the clog by hand, if you're handy. If not, ask a plumber.

Oven cleaners. Lye is also the active ingredient in many oven cleaners. Because lye is so dangerous, it's best to avoid lye-based oven cleaners, especially those in aerosol cans. While aerosols ensure that the material is evenly dispersed in your oven, they also are good at coating your skin, hair, and lungs with fine droplets that burn and irritate delicate tissues and that cause respiratory distress. As an alternative to using lye-based oven cleaners, mix up a thick gluey paste of baking soda and water and when the oven is cool, cover the spots with it. Let it sit for a bit—before it dries out, scrape up the spots or gently scrub them with steel wool. Rinse with a clean cloth dipped into a dilute solution of ¼ cup vinegar in a cup or two of water. It's pretty quick and not hard to do—and it makes the task much more pleasant than with lye-based cleaners that leave you gulping for fresh air while your eyes sting with harsh cleaner fumes.

The self-cleaning feature on your oven can also produce unhealthy fumes. It uses extreme heat to burn off the drippings in the oven, but it also manages to vaporize industrial oven coatings—not fumes you want to inhale!

Petroleum-based polyurethane floor and furniture finishes. These products contain several highly toxic substances, including toluene di-isocyanate (TDI). When inhaled, TDI fumes can cause airway sensitivity; if a person is re-exposed to TDI sometime in the future, it can cause a severe, acute, chemically induced asthma. Instead, use water-based polyurethane floor and furniture finishes, which are safer and less toxic. And always make sure your house is well ventilated when you apply polyurethane; air out the house for a few days afterward until the polyurethane fumes are not noticeable.

Paint removers. Most paint removers are very dangerous. Products containing methylene chloride are especially toxic and can cause severe blood and liver problems if their fumes are inhaled. If you need to use paint remover, choose products without methylene chloride. The California State Department of Public Health has been involved in a program to reduce worker death from methylene chloride. It recommends that, instead of methylene chloride strippers, strippers that are soy based or contain benzoyl alcohol or dibasic esters are preferred. However, these can produce eye, nose, throat, lung, and skin irritation. Anyone with asthma should not be exposed to these products. Keep in mind that you always need adequate ventilation with paint strippers and you will need to follow product instructions.

Mildew removers. Most mildew removers contain potent chemicals that can cause respiratory irritation and other adverse health effects. Check for safer mold and mildew removers on the Environmental Working Group's website www.ewg.org. Or try making your own mildew/mold remover—make a paste of baking soda and water and applying it to the affected area, such as bathtub grout. Scrub and rinse with a dilute solution of vinegar and water. Or try using 1% to 3% hydrogen peroxide. Make sure you test a small area with either product to be certain it won't cause damage to the tub surface or fabric that has the mildew stain.

Craft (airplane) glue. Most of the glues used to put together models contain substances that can be very hazardous to children. Solvents in some craft glues are neurotoxic chemicals that can damage a child's developing brain and nervous system and can even be lethal. In fact, each year children are brought to the emergency department with neurotoxicity related to glue sniffing (when kids intentionally sniff glue to get high).

But high levels can also occur when a child uses these products in a poorly ventilated room. Even a child using the glue as it was meant to be used—for building a model toy—can still experience toxic effects from the glue, such as dizziness or blurred vision, depending on the size of the room, how well it's ventilated, and how much glue is used. Our advice is to use nontoxic alternatives, such as wood or white glue, whenever possible. If the nontoxic glues won't work, use the smallest possible amount of craft glue in a well-ventilated room or, better still, outdoors, under close adult supervision. Air out the room frequently and have the child leave the room regularly to avoid continuous exposure to the glue's fumes.

Fingernail polish remover. Many polish removers contain acetone, a toxic solvent that vaporizes readily. Try a non-acetone product, which generally contains a solvent that doesn't vaporize as easily. Look for the words "acetone free" on the bottle's label. If you or your child must use an acetone product, do so in a well-ventilated room.

Also, don't let your child spend an extended period of time in a nail salon—where large quantities of acetone and other volatile and noxious solvents are used.

Hair spray contains lacquers and other ingredients that may be respiratory irritants to children. And using hair spray in a small, confined space, such as your bathroom, can build up the levels of irritants rapidly, especially if you are using an aerosol can. So choose products with non-aerosol containers and use them in a well-ventilated area.

Newly painted walls. Fresh paint emits solvents as it dries. Ventilate your house or apartment well for several days to a few weeks after painting to minimize the buildup of chemicals. Also, choose water-based paints, which generally have fewer toxic solvents than oil-based paints.

New furniture and rugs. New furniture and rugs can contain formaldehyde and other chemical solvents, which is what accounts for the "new" smell. Formaldehyde, however, is a potent carcinogen and respiratory toxin. Consider eco-friendly furniture and rugs, instead. But if you do bring home new furniture or rugs that contain formaldehyde or other chemical solvents, ventilate your house well every day for several days to several weeks to minimize the buildup of formaldehyde and other chemicals from these products. Washing out or airing cotton or synthetic rugs until the "new" smell disappears is a good idea. Do the same thing with new shower curtains or anything that is portable and has that "new" chemical smell— wash them and/or air them until the smell is gone.

Is wall-to-wall carpeting an allergen?

Wall-to-wall carpeting can generate lots of problems, from cradle to grave. New carpeting emits chemicals, such as formaldehyde, which are respiratory irritants. As new carpeting ages, it collects dust that can trigger allergies and asthma. Carpeting can also collect lead dust and other toxic materials brought into the home on peoples' shoes. The inevitable coffee and juice spills encourage mold to grow in the carpeting, which can cause everything from sneezing and eye irritation to shortness of breath.

You might think that shampooing your carpet would eliminate those problems, but rug shampoos actually contain toxic respiratory irritants. Studies by the National Institute for Occupational Safety and Health (NIOSH) have shown that the ingredients in rug shampoos can cause respiratory irritation and allergy symptoms, such as watering eyes. When shampooed carpet dries, the shampoo residue containing the toxic irritants becomes airborne. Once inhaled, the residue can cause shortness of breath and wheezing.

If you have wall-to-wall carpeting in your house, your best option is to replace all of it with machine-washable cotton or synthetic rugs. If you can replace only some of it, start with your child's room first.

Of course, replacing the carpeting may not be an option for you. In that case, frequently vacuum the carpeting using a vacuum with a HEPA filter, if you can. Establish a "no food or drink" rule in rooms with carpets. Air out the house often, especially on those bright, dry days when the wind can blow briskly through the house or apartment. And instead of using regular rug shampoos, try using the least toxic products available.

Does my pet pollute my home's air?

Dogs and cats shed fur and dander, both potent allergens. If your child has significant allergies or any type of wheezing or asthma, you shouldn't have a dog or cat that sheds allergens living in your house or coming into the house. Animal dander can trigger asthma attacks or cause uncomfortable allergy symptoms, such as red, itchy eyes and a runny nose. Some hypoallergenic breeds of cats and dogs generally do not cause exacerbations in children who are allergic to pets.

Do I need a mattress cover?

Yes. Pillows, mattresses, box springs, sheets, and blankets are all homes for dust mites—microscopic creatures that trigger allergies in many kids. And while you can wash sheets and blankets (something you should try to do weekly), you can't exactly stuff your whole bed into the washing machine.

What you can do, though, is cover both your child's mattress and box spring with a zippered, tightly woven, lightweight cloth (not plastic) cover, which is available online or in any home store. Avoid any product treated with "Microban" or that comes with claims that it protects against mold, mildew, or bacteria. This type of product usually contains triclosan, an endocrine-disrupting antimicrobial that can accumulate in children's bodies and cause chemical changes.

A tightly woven cloth mattress protector is also a possible protection from bedbugs, pests that can show up in any setting, regardless of conditions, in many parts of the world. Although these insects do not carry communicable diseases, they do bite, and they can be a nuisance to get rid of.

Are stuffed animals okay to have around?

In addition to invading your pillows and blankets, dust mites also make their home in the plush fur of the stuffed animals that kids love. If your child has significant allergies or any type of wheezing or asthma, nonwashable stuffed animals are off limits. Dusty stuffed animals can trigger an asthma attack or cause uncomfortable allergy symptoms, such as a runny nose or itchy eyes. And any time a child is exposed to dusty stuffed animals, his or her asthma attacks or allergic symptoms can actually become worse or more chronic.

If you want your child to breathe easy, make sure that any stuffed animals your child collects are washable—and then throw them in the washing machine once a week. If your child doesn't have allergies or has only rare bouts of milder allergies and no regular bouts of wheezing, you can be a bit more relaxed about nonwashable stuffed animals. However, you should be aware that dust in the stuffed animals might contribute to your child's occasional misery. And continual exposure to allergens can make a mild case of allergies worse. If you child's bouts with allergies increase or he starts wheezing more often, you should reconsider the decision to let him have nonwashable stuffed animals.

7

ENDOCRINE DISRUPTORS
IN THE HOME

Endocrine disruptors are man-made chemicals that can hack the body's chemical-based signaling system—the endocrine system.

The endocrine system is the network of glands that regulate growth and development in children, reproduction in young adults, and aging in older adults. The endocrine system includes the pituitary, called the "master gland" because it regulates the other glands in the body, the thyroid, the pancreas, the adrenals, the ovaries in girls and women, and the testes in boys and men.

Endocrine glands send signals to cells and organs throughout the body by releasing tiny amounts of extremely powerful chemicals—hormones—into the blood. These hormones trigger actions within cells. Thus, in an emergency, the adrenals release adrenaline (epinephrine), which enables us to fight an enemy or to run swiftly away from danger. The thyroid releases thyroid hormone—thyroxine—which regulates metabolism and is critical for brain development in infants. Hormones released by the ovaries—estrogens—and from the testes—androgens—regulate the timing of puberty and are essential for reproduction.

Many manufactured chemicals developed in recent decades and placed in consumer products are now known to interfere with the action of natural hormones. These chemicals are called *endocrine disruptors*. They can cause disease and disrupt normal development in children by interfering with the action of naturally occurring hormones—including growth hormones, estrogens, testosterone, insulin, and thyroid hormone.

Millions of pounds of endocrine-disrupting chemicals are manufactured each year in the United States for use in household plastics, soaps, shampoos, cosmetics, air fresheners, cleaning products, motor fuel, furniture flame-proofing, pesticides, stain-repellant sprays, metal can linings, tableware, and medical equipment. As shown in national surveys conducted by the Centers for Disease Control and Prevention (CDC), these chemicals are routinely detected in the bodies and blood levels of most Americans.

What are the most common endocrine disruptors?

Bisphenol A, known commonly as BPA, is a manufactured chemical produced in large quantities primarily for use in epoxy resins and polycarbonate plastics. Polycarbonate plastics are widely used in food and beverage packaging, including water bottles and infant bottles, linings of metal food cans, impact-resistant safety equipment, compact discs, and medical devices. Epoxy resins are used as lacquer coating in metal products, such as bottle tops, food cans, and pipes that supply drinking water. BPA is also used in dental sealants and composites, as well as in some thermal papers used for cash register and credit card receipts.

BPA can leach into food from the epoxy resins used to line food cans and from polycarbonate consumer products, such as drinking water bottles. The primary source of most daily exposure to BPA is believed to be through the diet.

Phthalates are oily, liquid chemicals used to make rigid plastics soft and flexible. They are found in a wide range of both industrial and consumer products, such as shower curtains, intravenous bags, vinyl, inks, floor tiles, and, until the late 20th century, in infants' nipples and pacifiers. Products made with PVC, such as plastic food wrap, children's toys, and PVC pipe, also contain phthalates.

Phthalates are used to help products retain their color and scent. They can be found in shampoos, cosmetics, air fresheners, and household cleaners. Products that list "fragrance" as an ingredient may include phthalates.

Phthalates are powerful endocrine disruptors. Prenatal exposure to phthalates is associated with disrupted development of the brain and reproductive organs. The consequence is changes in behavior in boys and girls and feminization of the reproductive organs in boys.

Organophosphate insecticides are synthetic chemicals originally developed for chemical warfare during World War II. The chemical weapon sarin is an organophosphate. Today, organophosphates are among the pesticides most widely used for the extermination of crawling household insects and in outdoor sprays to keep flying insects out of the yard. Among the widely used organophosphate pesticides are malathion, diazinon, and chlorpyrifos.

Organophosphate pesticides are now known to be toxic to the brain and nervous system as well as endocrine disruptors. Prenatal exposure to these chemicals have been linked to abnormalities in brain development in infants. They may also increase the risk of obesity and diabetes.

Polychlorinated biphenyls (PCBs) are extremely stable, nonflammable, oily chemicals that resist heat. They have been used extensively as insulators, flame retardants, stabilizers, sealants, and adhesives. They were used in the ballasts of fluorescent light fixtures, caulking, linoleum, ceiling tiles, and wood varnish. Although PCBs are no longer manufactured or distributed in most countries, many PCB-containing products developed prior to the PCB ban are still in use. People continue to be exposed to PCBs from consumption of fish, meat, and dairy products, because PCBs are persistent in the environment and move up the food chain, or bioaccumulate. For example, when many small fish with PCBs are eaten by larger fish, all of the PCBs go into the larger fish and stay there until they are consumed by something "higher" on the food chain, including humans, depositing all of the collected PCBs into our bodies.

PCBs are endocrine disruptors. Exposures in early life and especially prenatally are linked to developmental disabilities, learning disabilities, memory impairment, and psychomotor dysfunction.

Brominated flame retardants, which have the chemical name polybrominated diphenyl ethers (PDBEs), are chemical that are very similar to PCBs. PDBEs are used extensively in consumer products, such as computers, curtains, furniture, and carpets, as well as in industrial products, especially in plastics and textiles.

Like PCBs, brominated flame retardants are persistent in the environment. A growing body of evidence indicates that PDBEs are endocrine disruptors that are dangerous to humans and especially to infants and young children. Prenatal exposures to PBDEs are linked to lowered IQ in children and to disruption of behavior.

In the United States, PDBEs continue to be used as flame retardants in mattresses and furniture, and PDBE levels in the environment and in people continue to grow, doubling every two to five years. By contrast, in Sweden, where PDBEs have been banned, the PDBE levels in people have dropped dramatically. Some states in the United States, most notably California, Oregon, Ilinois, Michigan, and Vermont have enacted bans on brominated flame retardants.

Are there other chemicals in commercial use that are endocrine disruptors?

Currently, there are no standard tests to determine if a particular substance is an endocrine disruptor. Both the Clean Water Act and the Food Quality Protection Act (1996) required the Environmental Protection Agency (EPA) to develop test methods.

Researchers are looking into some additional chemicals widely used in the production of household products to determine whether these chemicals are endocrine disruptors. Results of the studies will enable scientists to hone in on dangerous endocrine disruptors that should be removed from the marketplace.

Although not all the information is in, some chemicals of current concern include:

Glycol ethers, which are solvents that can be found in some paint, cleaning products, brake fluids, and some cosmetics. They are linked with decreased fertility in painters and may damage the fertility of an unborn child, according to the European Union.

Parabens, which are common additives to beauty and cosmetic products. They are a family of compounds coming under increased scrutiny and concern as endocrine disruptors. Found in shampoos, conditioners, deodorants, cleansers, facial scrubs, eye makeup, and lotions, they are preservatives that discourage the growth of microbes. Current research centers on their possible links to breast cancer.

So do plastics contain endocrine disruptors?

Many plastics are known to contain endocrine disruptors. Since it is difficult to imagine avoiding all plastic consumer products, it is useful to have some ways to make using plastics a bit safer.

Plastic food containers are often labeled on the bottom with a plastic recycling code, indicating the type of plastic used in the product. Here are the labels deciphered:

#1 PET (polyethylene terephthalate)
#2 HDPE (high density polyethylene)
#3 PVC (polyvinylchloride)
#4 LDPE (low density polyethylene)
#5 PP (polypropylene)

#6 PS (polystyrene)

#7 Other (often polycarbonate)

The safer plastics are those made with polyethylene (#1), but it is not recommended that #1 plastic be reused.

The saying, "5, 4, 1, or 2. All the rest are bad for you!" may help you choose the safer plastics when you when do your household and grocery shopping.

Children's toys should be checked for plastic components as well, with the same guidelines applied as above. Many toys are made of polyvinylchloride (PVC) and should be avoided.

Can I microwave foods in plastic containers or with plastic wrap?

No, it's not a good idea to microwave foods in plastic containers or covered with plastic wrap.

New plastic food containers and food wraps contain chemicals called plasticizers, which provide softness and flexibility. Plasticizers include phthalates and bisphenol A (BPA), both of which are endocrine disruptors. But plasticizers don't stay in the plastic wrap or plastic container, especially if the wrap or container is subjected to extreme conditions, such as being heated in the microwave oven. Instead, they are released into the food where they find their way into our bodies through inhalation or ingestion.

You can minimize the amounts of harmful chemicals leaching into your food and air from plastic containers by using stable containers like glass, porcelain, or stainless steel for cooking and storing food.

Do water bottles contain endocrine disruptors?

Plastic water bottles and drinks packaged in plastic containers may also contain the same endocrine disruptors as the cooking plastics discussed above, and the water or drink stored in the plastic bottles may contain minute quantities of chemicals used in manufacturer of the plastic. Stainless steel water bottles offer the best guarantee of not ingesting chemicals leached from a portable drinking container.

Is cold water safer than hot water for cooking and drinking?

Yes. Hot water can leach more chemicals from household plumbing than cold water, so using cold water for drinking, cooking, and reconstituting baby formula reduces the risk of ingesting chemicals. Cold water that has been sitting in your household pipes for hours can also leach minute quantities of lead and other chemicals from your household plumbing, so letting the tap run for 30 seconds before you fill the pan or teapot helps mitigate exposure, too. (The water that is run during the 30 seconds need not be discarded—it can be used for watering plants or other uses not involving human consumption.)

Are all baby bottles safe?

Until well into the 21st century, plastic baby bottles made of polycarbonates were a major source of exposure of countless infants to bisphenol A (BPA), a potent endocrine disruptor. Concerned parents, given the information that BPA is dangerous, have undertaken grassroots campaigns to get the BPA out of baby bottles and other plastics used in families with children. Many manufacturers responded to these concerns and voluntarily eliminated BPA from many of their products. Advertising campaigns were then built around the products' "BPA-free" composition—a tribute to the resiliency and strength of the marketplace in responding to consumer concerns.

However, there is still BPA in some products, including some baby bottles. Furthermore, some of the chemicals that manufacturers have used in place of BPA include bisphenol S (BPS), which, as its name implies, is a close cousin to BPA and may also be an endocrine disruptor.

Until legislation or consumer pressure succeeds in uniform removal of BPA and BPS from all baby products, glass bottles with silicone nipples remain the safer alternative to plastic baby bottles. The risk of breakage from heavy-duty glass bottles is relatively low.

Why do we recommend silicone for nipples and pacifiers?

The nipples on baby bottles and pacifiers need to be soft and flexible in order to do what they're supposed to do. The softness and flexibility of many pacifiers and nipples on the market are ensured in manufacture through the addition of plasticizers, such as phthalates. Phthalates are endocrine-disrupting chemicals.

Silicone is naturally soft and does not require plasticizers during manufacture.

What types of food packaging contain endocrine disruptors?

The epoxy lining of canned foods often contains BPA, a known endocrine disruptor. The epoxy lining is used to make sure that the contents of the can do not react with the can itself. Some manufacturers are exploring ways of substituting safer materials in the liners of canned foods, but for now, the surest method of minimizing this risk is to purchase BPA-free canned food—or to buy fresh food and bypass the packaging altogether.

Does cookware contain endocrine disruptors?

Some nonstick cookware contains endocrine-disrupting chemicals known as PFCs (perfluorinated chemicals). PFCs can leach or rub off into foods through normal cooking processes involving stirring and serving.

However, PFCs are extremely stable chemical compounds that that don't break down in the environment or in landfills and will be with us indefinitely. Nearly every one of us has minute traces of these chemicals in our bodies already. They are in the bodies of today's children and will be in the bodies of future generations' children, too.

Some PFCs are now known to be endocrine disruptors. They have been linked to low birth weight, male fertility problems, thyroid disease, kidney disease, and high cholesterol. Other PFCs have incomplete test data.

Are there furniture and carpet components that are toxic?

The chemicals used to promote stain resistance in commercial fabrics—including upholstery and carpeting—are PFCs (perfluorinated chemicals). Persistent in the environment, these chemicals are endocrine disruptors that don't break down in landfills. Many couches, chairs and other stuffed furniture as well as some carpets and widow curtains contain highly hazardous flame retardant chemicals—see next paragraph.

Do flame retardants pose the same threats as stain repellants?

Both flame retardants and stain repellants contain endocrine disruptors. Flame-retardant chemicals are present in most consumer goods, including computers, televisions, mobile phones, automotive equipment, construction materials, polyurethane foam mattresses, cushions, upholstered furniture, carpets, and draperies. Flame retardants all contain chemicals called PBDEs (polybrominated diphenyl ethers), which until a generation ago were also incorporated into children's pajamas. At first glance, making anything resistant to fire sounds like a great idea. But closer inspection tells a different story.

PBDEs have a chemical structure similar to PCBs, a known endocrine disruptor. Prenatal exposures are especially concerning and can result in lowered IQ and behavioral problems. Like PCBs, PBDEs are ubiquitous and persistent in the environment and are found in ever-increasing amounts in our bodies. PBDEs are easily shed from products since they are not chemically bound to the product structure.

Parents can minimize children's exposure to flame retardants by looking for PBDE-free product labels when choosing mattresses and furnishings. Alternatives to PBDEs are less readily available in other products and will remain so barring new legislation.

Are endocrine disruptors present in soaps?

Some soaps, especially those containing fragrance or antimicrobial agents, may contain endocrine disruptors.

Frequent hand washing with soap and water remains the best overall method to fight the spread of illness and disease; when unavailable, use a hand-sanitizer containing at least 60% alcohol. These products are very effective for most germs, but may be less effective in removing toxins or germs from obviously dirty hands. It might seem logical that using the strongest antimicrobial soap would be the best and most effective choice. But it isn't.

Here's why you should not use antimicrobial soap:

There is no evidence that antimicrobial soaps are any better than soap and water.

In September, 2016, the US Food and Drug Administration (FDA) ruled that antimicrobial cleaners are no more effective than soap and water in preventing the spread of germs—and that antimicrobial products can no longer be marketed in bar soaps, foams, and liquid hand-washing gels, shampoos, and body washes.

The antimicrobial chemicals used in these products, triclosan and triclocarban, are persistent environmental pollutants.

With everything that goes down the drain, from soap bubbles to discarded or excreted prescription medications, there is a good chance some of it will come back to plague us through contamination of our water and food.

What goes down the drain enters the waste stream and passes through the wastewater treatment plant before being discharged into the environment. Some substances are persistent enough to make the journey through the treatment plant, down the river, and into the clouds that bring rain to farms and drinking water reservoirs. These chemicals come back to haunt us in our food and water and are called persistent environmental pollutants (POPs).

The CDC has found that triclosan is present in the urine of 75% of the US population, with concentrations that have increased by 50% since 2004.

Triclosan and triclocarban are endocrine disruptors.

These antimicrobial endocrine disruptors are already present in the bodies of most of the American population. Like other endocrine disruptors in our bodies, they may be busy right now, meddling with our cells, pretending to be natural hormones. As endocrine mimics, they gain access to our cells and can interfere with natural hormones' roles in the control of daily cell processes, in growth and development of infants and children, in the timing of adolescence and sexual maturation, and in aging. New research shows that the effects of endocrine-disrupting chemicals can be multigenerational; in other words, the damaging effects of the chemicals can be passed through our genes to future generations.

Do air fresheners contain endocrine disruptors?

Yes. Products used to promote pleasant odors generally contain phthalates, which are known endocrine disruptors. Plug-in air fresheners produce especially high levels of these toxic compounds.

So does perfume contain endocrine disruptors, too? What about cosmetics?

Some perfumes and cosmetic products do contain phthalates, parabens, or glycol ether, which are all known endocrine disruptors. However, because the ingredients in cosmetic products are not always readily discernible from their labels, it can be difficult for consumers to know what chemicals they're applying to their skin.

The Environmental Working Group (www.ewg.org), a nonprofit organization based in the United States, is compiling an extensive database called Skin Deep (http://www.ewg.org/skindeep/)—of cosmetic and beauty products available to the consumer, highlighting what is known about each listed ingredient in the product. Although the database is very much a work in progress, it currently highlights the fact that scant information is available about many ingredients and chemicals we apply to our skin in the name of health and beauty. As researchers develop more information on the health and safety of ingredients used in these products, a clearer picture should emerge about which products should be avoided when purchasing cosmetics.

8

PESTICIDES AND HERBICIDES

Pesticides are chemicals designed to kill living organisms They are used to protect against or destroy pests—rodents, insects, fungi, weeds and other living interlopers. Herbicides are a type of pesticide that kills unwanted plant life—what the language of today's lawn and garden culture terms "weeds." The use of these substances in commercial farming and private homes is so widespread (and the substances' chemical compositions so varied) that it warrants a discussion of their roles in childhood chemical exposures. A related discussion occurs in Chapter 9, on food, but it's equally important to understand the exposures that occur in the name of lawn care and pest remediation.

What's wrong with pesticides?

Pesticides offer what seems to be a quick and easy solution to a problem—protection against, or extermination of living pests that target plants or homes. But pesticide use carries unwanted side effects and pesticide use often creates new problems.

Pesticides lack precision—in addition to killing pests, they also kill beneficial insects, birds, and animals, and they have harmful effects on humans. Also pesticides can prompt adaptations in the organisms they target, thereby making the organisms stronger than they were previously. For example, an insecticide may wipe out only the weaker bugs; the stronger ones will regroup, survive, and multiply, stronger than they were before. Widespread use of chemical herbicides has led to the emergence of herbicide-resistant weeds. Since pesticides don't distinguish between helpful organisms and harmful organisms, when you're out spraying your vegetable or flower garden, you're killing off all the butterflies, bees, beetles, and other helpful insects that are necessary for pollination and that also prey on the bad bugs. And while you're dosing bugs indoors or outdoors with pesticides, you're exposing your children to toxic chemicals that can harm their health.

What are organophosphate pesticides?

Organophosphates are a class of pesticides that, until the 21st century, were among the most widely used pesticides available. They are used in commercial and home settings to kill insects and other intrusive bugs, and they are extremely toxic, even life-threatening. People have been poisoned by organophosphates from skin contact, by breathing the vapors, or by accidental ingestion. The war gas sarin, used in the infamous 1995 Tokyo Subway Attack is an member of the organophosphate family. Symptoms of serious, high-dose organophosphate exposure include blurred vision, abdominal pain, increased salivation, sweating, irritability, nausea, vomiting, muscle spasms, mental confusion, and seizures. But exposures to orthophosphates at levels too low to produce symptoms can also cause harm, especially to children. Exposures to some organophosphates during pregnancy have been linked to low birth weight, smaller head circumference, and developmental delays in children exposed prenatally.

One well-known organophosphate, chlorpyrifos (Dursban), was widely used until 2001 as a pesticide for roach control in apartment buildings, and as a home and garden pesticide to kill fleas, ticks, bees, wasps, hornets, termites, and roaches. In 2001, it was banned from home use in an effort to reduce children's exposure to it. Chlorpyrifos is still widely used in agriculture; as a result, its residues are measurable on a variety of fruits and vegetables in grocery stores. Efforts to remove chlorpyrifos from the marketplace continue to be blocked by the chemical industry and in March 2017 the current EPA Administrator delayed implementation of regulations that would further limit its use.

According to surveys done by the Centers for Disease Control and Prevention (CDC), over 90% of the population of the United States has measurable amounts of chlorpyrifos in their bodies. It can even be found in samples of Arctic ice. Chlorpyrifos is also a relatively persistent pollutant in the environment and even though the use of this pesticide has been greatly curtailed, children and their families continue to be exposed.

Chlorpyrifos is a known to be toxic to the developing human brain. Prenatal exposure to chlorpyrifos has been documented in multiple studies to reduce IQ, shorten attention span, and cause behavioral problems in infants. When they are exposed to chlorpyrifos prenatally, babies are also at risk of having small heads at birth—a measure of slowed brain growth seen also in babies exposed prenatally to Zika virus. MRI studies of 7- and 8-year-old children who were exposed to chlorpyrifos before birth show changes in brain anatomy and function.

Other organophosphate pesticides still available in the marketplace include diazinon and malathion. A related pesticide, carbaryl (Sevin), is also available for home use. These other organophospahates have not been studied as extensively as chlorpyrifos but act through many of the same chemical mechanisms and may therefore be anticipated to have similar toxic effects.

Chlorpyrifos and other organophosphate pesticides, even when used according to the manufacturer's directions indoors, can accumulate on rugs and children's toys, providing an ongoing exposure to these toxic chemicals.

Is pesticide use increasing or decreasing?

Use of some older pesticides is decreasing, but at the same time use of certain classes of pesticides, especially newer pesticides is increasing.

Neonicotinoid insecticides are a class of chemicals known to be toxic to the nervous system whose use is increasing rapidly. One neonicotinoid, imidacloprid, introduced only about 20 years ago, is now widely used in the world. Neonicotinoids have been implicated in the collapse of bee colonies worldwide—they act on bees by damaging their brains and nervous systems and may be responsible for impairing their ability to navigate. The resulting devastation to food crops and to ecosystems has the potential to be enormous, given bee colonies' essential role in the pollination of crops. European countries are beginning to ban or severely restrict the use of neonicotinoids. Despite the neonicotinoids' wide use, almost nothing is known about their human health effects. But because these chemicals are known to be neurotoxic to insects, there are serious unanswered questions about their possible effects on humans, and especially on children.

The herbicide glyphosate, marketed under the trade name Roundup, is another pesticide whose use is increasing rapidly. Glyphosate is used extensively in agriculture to kill weeds in the production of genetically modified crops—corn, soybeans, and sugar beets. It is available also for home and garden applications. Its use has increased by 2,500% in the past 25 years. The World Health Organization has recently concluded that glyphosate is a probable human carcinogen a chemical judged probably capable of causing cancer in humans.

Are there safe, effective ways to get rid of pests without using pesticides?

Yes. A technique known as *integrated pest management* (IPM) is a common-sense approach to choosing the least toxic method of controlling pests. IPM uses chemical intervention only as a last line of defense.

IPM focuses on taking away the sources of food, water, and shelter for pests. This approach can establish a sustainable solution to the problem, rather than a temporary one or one that brings about larger problems. Nonchemical controls are preferentially used. For example, using an enclosed mousetrap to control rodents is better than using rodent poisons, which are toxic to children. Rather than using a pesticide spray to control insects, IPM would choose a sticky trap instead.

I am using an exterminator. What can I do to minimize chemical exposure from pesticides?

Here are things to consider if you are considering using an exterminator:

Choose only an exterminator who uses IPM techniques and ask for details about what IPM techniques he uses. Ask the exterminator how he would assess your problem and what steps he would take to solve it. Is his answer consistent with IPM techniques?

Make sure the exterminator is a certified pesticide applicator. Most states require pesticide applicators to be certified. Ask to see proof.

If the exterminator suggests using pesticides, ask about the pesticides he will use. Ask for an MSDS (material data safety sheet) on every pesticide that would be used to solve your problem. The MSDS is a fact sheet that provides the chemical name of the pesticide, as well as information about its toxicity and potential health effects. Be wary if you don't get specific, detailed information about the product the exterminator will use. The product name is not sufficient. Also remember that "completely safe" pesticides don't exist. Use due diligence in researching the pesticide before agreeing to pesticide application.

Ask what safer alternatives he can offer. A pesticide professional who uses IPM should be able show you ways of preventing pest problems without resorting to pesticides time and time again.

Ask how often extermination will be necessary. The right answer is that regular inspections will be done and pesticides will be applied only when a demonstrated pest problem exists that cannot be solved by other means. Committing to monthly maintenance or any other system that uses regular applications of pesticide "to prevent the problem from recurring" is not recommended.

Are lawn chemicals toxic?

Yes, many are toxic. Dozens of chemicals are used for lawn beautification in the United States, and they include carcinogens, endocrine disruptors, and substances known to damage other systems of the body. CDC surveys have found that these substances are present in the bodies of most Americans.

I don't use lawn chemicals or other pesticides. How is it possible that my household is still exposed to these toxic chemicals?

Consider this troubling problem: your windows are open and your children are playing in the backyard with their toys scattered everywhere. A green-and-white truck pulls up in front of your next-door neighbor's house and a lawn maintenance worker in a crisp white uniform unrolls a hose from the truck and starts spraying toxic materials on the lawn next door. A fine chemical mist coats the toys in the yard and your kids. The children also inhale the noxious fumes.

The term for what you are seeing here is *pesticide drift*— that is, pesticides have wafted from the area where they are being applied into your backyard or from a farmer's field into a school playground. Pesticide drift can expose households to toxic materials without their knowledge. It can come from a neighbor's yard or a nearby farmer's field, or just from wearing pesticide-contaminated shoes in the house. Studies have shown that some widely used pesticides can remain where they were sprayed for weeks after initial spraying. Other studies show that pesticides are easily tracked into the house, exposing the children who play on the floor.

Here are a few simple steps to protect from this hazard.

Conduct some neighborly negotiations to try to remedy the problem. Find out what chemicals are being used on the neighbor's property and explain your concern about the pesticides' spreading into your yard and harming your children. You might want to bring along some educational materials on the topic—including this book. Perhaps also have available the name of a company that uses nontoxic products that you can steer the neighbors to.

Contact your local health department or environmental protection agency. Ask if there are any laws or regulations in your area regulating pesticide drift. Many cities and towns in Canada and the United States now have such laws.

Get your neighbors together to address the problem. Some towns have laws that require neighbors to be notified 48 hours in advance of the application of pesticides on adjoining properties. If you know at least 48 hours in advance, you'll have time to close your windows, bring in the children's toys, and keep the children indoors. And if there is no local law, consider working with your neighbors and your elected officials to get one passed.

How can I tell if a yard has been treated with pesticides?

Even if you don't use pesticides on your own lawn, you've probably noticed how many of your neighbors' lawns display "pesticide flags."

Pesticide flags are the required notices to passers-by to stay off the grass for 24 hours because pesticide has been applied to the lawn. But dogs and children probably don't observe the pesticide flags, and many of the flags seem to stay up for weeks or longer, so it is difficult to know which warnings are current and which have expired. The pesticide treatment flags on the lawns tell you something else—they give you an idea how many neighbors are using pesticides to keep their grass looking nice. This is called "cosmetic" pesticide use.

Some localities have begun to pass laws against cosmetic pesticide use. The City Council of Takoma Park, Maryland, and the Province of Ontario, Canada passed laws to restrict the cosmetic use of pesticides on public and private properties. These laws reduce pesticide exposures and also help to prevent pesticide drift and pesticide migration from treated properties to untreated properties.

Pesticides are chemicals that have been devised to kill pests. Insecticides kill insects by disrupting an insect's neurological system—a basic biological system that we humans also have. Moreover, insect brains and human brains share many of the same enzyme systems. Is it reasonable to think that we are immune to such toxins?

Keep your children and pets safe by keeping them away from pesticide-treated lawns. Better yet, encourage your neighbors to use the least toxic materials available to control lawn problems and to rethink their attachment to a weed-free monoculture lawn. A few dandelions can be a beautiful sign that people are not using toxic chemicals to the detriment of people and the environment.

How can I have a nice lawn without chemical fertilizers and pesticides?

The safer approach to a nice, green lawn—give or take a dandelion or two—works like this:

Plant the right grass for your region of the country. Native plants grow the best in any environment. Nature has already made the selection about what grows best— don't go to war with nature. Find out what types of grass grow best in your region by contacting your local cooperative extension office, a service of the United States Department of Agriculture.

Adjust your lawn mower blade to its highest setting. Longer blades of grass will enable the grass to develop stronger root systems and compete better with weeds. Taller grass also protects the root system of the grass by shading the roots from the harsh rays of the sun. On dry days, the longer blades help the root system maintain some moisture, and therefore they really help to minimize the lawn's need for extra water.

Leave your grass clippings on the lawn. When grass clippings break down, they add valuable nitrogen to the soil, which in turn creates a healthy self-fertilized lawn. A mulching mower will help the process move along a little faster. In the spring, give the lawn a brisk raking to remove any remaining thatch and allow the baby grass blades to get an early start.

Use nontoxic methods of weed control for weeds you can't live with. Hand weeding can be a relaxing and satisfying excuse for spending an hour outdoors on a nice day. Don't keep count of how many are still left—learn to make peace with your lawn.

To discourage broadleaf weeds from taking over the lawn, apply corn gluten to the lawn at the same time that the forsythia is blooming. Corn gluten is a natural, pre-emergent weed controller and is readily available in many garden stores and online. For well-established broadleaf weeds, hand weeding is the best nontoxic control.

Replace some of the lawn with a small rock or native plant garden. Your local library will have designs for small garden areas to suit any style of house. Planting a small rock garden with native plants can cut down on lawn watering needs. Find native plants that like the location you have chosen and they will thrive with little care.

My home has termites. How bad are the various options for extermination in terms of toxicity?

Termites have their own rightful place in world's ecosystem (they help turn fallen timber and wood debris into sawdust that then enters the cycle of renewal and rebirth), but they can also become household pests capable of great damage to homes if they infest the wood.

Traditional treatments for termite infestation use highly toxic chemicals:

Chlordane, a highly toxic chlorinated chemical, was used for decades as the chemical of choice for termite control. Exterminators drilled holes around the foundation of a house and filled the holes with the pesticide. The resulting levels of chlordane in homes were high enough to contaminate the homes and create long-term health concerns, including cancer. Chlordane was banned by the Environmental Protection Agency (EPA) in 1988, but it was still found at high levels in some treated homes 35 years later. The CDC's Fourth National Report on Human Exposure to Environmental Chemicals showed that as of January 2017, the US population continued to have measurable amounts of chlordane in their bodies.

Chlorpyrifos, an organophosphate pesticide, was the first choice for use against termites by most commercial exterminators until it was phased out by the EPA in 2005 because of its well-documented hazards to human health, especially to the brains of infants and children. Other chemicals, some with even more concerning toxic properties, have taken its place.

Many current termite treatments also use toxic pesticides. According to the EPA, the most common pesticide mixtures used today to kill termites include one or more of the following pesticides:

Acetamiprid is a neonicotinoid, a new type of insecticide that may be implicated in the worldwide collapse of honeybee populations. Definitive studies of its effects on long-term human health have yet to be done, but the chemical is of great concern because it acts by targeting the nervous system.

Bifenthrin is a synthetic pyrethroid, a class of widely used pesticides with toxicity to aquatic life. Some studies show pyrethroid pesticides to be endocrine disruptors in aquatic wildlife.

Chlorantraniliprole belongs to a new class of pesticides, anthranilic diamides. Definitive studies on its effects on long-term human health have yet to be done.

Chlorfenapyr is a moderately toxic pyrrole, a relatively new class of chemicals, that is highly toxic to bees and aquatic wildlife.

Cyfluthrin, cypermethrin, and **esfenvalerate** are also synthetic pyrethroids.

Fipronil is a pesticide in the pheynypyrazole family and is classified as a possible human carcinogen by the EPA. Animal studies have shown that fipronil can affect the ability of rats to produce offspring and that it delays development of the offspring.

Imidacloprid is a neonicotinoid, a class of insecticides that target the insect's nervous system. Some animal studies show reproductive effects, including reduced bone growth in offspring. Although imidacloprid is widespread in the environment, definitive studies on its effects on long-term human health have yet to be done.

Permethrin is a pyrethroid and is highly toxic to fish and aquatic animals, bees, and other beneficial insects. The EPA has classified it as likely to be carcinogenic to humans.

But there are some less toxic -options for killing termites:

Extreme cold. Exterminators inject liquid nitrogen into the walls of your home where termites have established their colonies. A big advantage of this method is that liquid nitrogen can reach termites in otherwise inaccessible areas.

Electrocution. Termites are electrocuted with a device that releases current through a probe that the exterminator runs over the surface of the wood.

Diatomaceous earth. This material kills termites by eroding their outer shell, causing them to dry up.

Biological controls. Beneficial nematodes (microscopic wormlike creatures) are mixed with water and injected into the soil around your home. Once in the soil, the nematodes seek out and kill the termites.

My home has roaches. Are nontoxic extermination options available?

Roaches can show up in homes in all parts of the country, no matter how clean your house is, although they are most likely to appear in urban or apartment housing, where many dwelling units occupy a small area. Worse than the mere sight of them, roach droppings can trigger asthma and allergies in kids.

Roach killers are toxic to the insect's brain and nervous system, and they can also damage the brains and nervous systems of small children. Some of these pesticides are also allergens and in some people, asthma attacks follow the use of this type of pesticide. As more research links children, pesticides, and asthma, the best bet is to walk on the safe side and to avoid using chemical pesticides.

To get rid of roaches in a safe, nontoxic way, try some or all of the following tactics to deny them food, water, and shelter—the integrated pest management approach described earlier:

Seal cracks and crevices. The most important thing you can do is to seal cracks and crevices in the walls, floors, and corners where the walls and floor meet; these can serve as secret hideaways for roaches and enable them to move from room to room without you noticing them. You can fill the small cracks with caulking compound, the way you fill the seams between the tile and bathtub. Fill larger cracks with wood shims and then caulk. Choose a non-toxic caulk for indoor use. Make sure you check under the sinks and fill in the cracks and crevices between the plumbing and the floor or walls—these are easy ways for roaches to get from one floor to another. Sealing the cracks will also help limit access by mice, should that ever be a problem for you.

Set out glue traps. Place the traps wherever you have seen roaches. Remove and replace them as they do their job.

Enforce the "no food in the bedroom" rule. Food attracts roaches, so confine the cookies and pizza crumbs to the kitchen and dining areas, where you can easily sweep them up. Keeping the children's rooms off limits for food will minimize the likelihood that roaches will settle there and trigger allergies while the children sleep.

Dry the kitchen before bedtime. Roaches like water sources and consider damp sponges and wet dishes left in the sink an open invitation to stop by. So dry those dishes and put the wet sponge in a plastic bag. Before storing a sponge overnight, make sure you wash it thoroughly with hot, soapy water. Wash it again in the morning before using it, to minimize the buildup of germs. You can also stick your sponge in the dishwasher and wash it along with the dishes to keep it clean and fresh.

Clean up dark corners. Grease and crumbs that accumulate in hard-to-reach places can support entire families of roaches. So periodically clean up food residue from under the refrigerator, behind the stove, and in any other out-of-the-way nooks and crannies in your kitchen.

Do most flea and tick collars on pets contain toxic chemicals?

Yes. Many commercially available tick collars offer months of flea and tick control, but they come with warnings to humans not to get dust from the collar or the collar itself in their mouths. Directions suggest preventing the collar from coming in contact with skin, eyes, or clothing. This could present a difficulty for a giggling toddler or young child wrestling with his best friend, the family dog.

Clearly, a tick collar with a pesticide that lasts for months is not a good choice for a household trying to avoid chemical toxicity. Luckily there are some good alternatives. There is an oral medicine available from veterinarians for flea protection and a good vaccine for dogs against Lyme disease. There are also tick collars with natural herbal remedies—talk it over with your veterinarian to see what's best. Finally, remember to avoid flea and tick control shampoo for dogs, too. If it kills ticks and fleas, it's probably not good for kids either.

Fleas can carry heartworm, a devastating illness in dogs, and ticks can carry Lyme disease. A tick bite can spread Lyme Disease to whoever is bitten–you, your child or your dog. So, while some manner of control is necessary, the least toxic intervention is optimal.

9

FOOD

The food system in the United States has plenty of shortcomings, not the least being that the most readily available food is generally the least healthy. Chemicals in our food are not discussed as they should be, and this chapter provides guidance on navigating the food–chemical environment. It begins where the last chapter left off, with pesticides.

Which foods are the most likely to contain toxic pesticide residues?

Fruits and vegetables are directly treated with pesticides, sometimes only days or hours before being shipped to market, and the pesticide chemicals are likely to remain present in or on the fruits and vegetables in large amounts while the foods await purchase on grocery store shelves. In the 1993 landmark report, *Pesticides in the Diets of Infants and Children*, the National Academy of Sciences expressed concern that the residual levels of pesticides found on produce may affect children's health and development. Researchers today have found that even minuscule amounts of pesticides can interfere with a child's brain or with the hormones that regulate growth and development. As the list of chemicals that can harm the developing infant and child continues to expand, parents are encouraged to do what they can to minimize their child's exposure to pesticide residues on fruits and vegetables. Here are some strategies that will help.

Use certified-organic produce when possible. The term "organic" is tightly regulated, and organic produce is grown without any pesticides, herbicides, or fertilizers. Because organic food is grown without chemicals, it's free of the toxic pesticide residues present on "traditionally grown" produce that is raised with the use of chemicals and pesticides. In order for fruits and vegetables to be labeled "organic," they must meet minimum criteria established by the federal government, allowing them to be labeled "certified organic." (Note: Food marketers have gotten creative with their use of other unregulated, meaningless terms such as **natural** or **homegrown**. While it's not foolproof, looking for the "USDA Organic" green label on foods is the best practice in the United States.)

Limit quantities of imported produce. Although most of the fruits and vegetables grown in the United States are treated with pesticide, the federal government has outlawed the use of many of the most dangerous pesticides, such as DDT, because of their long-term toxic effects. Unfortunately, chemical manufacturers have found a market for many of the banned chemicals in countries with less restrictive laws. Growers in countries outside of the United States use these toxic pesticides on fruits and vegetables that are then exported to the United States. Although the federal government regulates produce imported into the United States, regulation is imperfect and there is no doubt that traces of the banned pesticides manage to get into our food supply, in part due to lax enforcement of the bans at ports of entry.

The best way to tell whether fruits or vegetables are imported is to check the label. If you can't tell from the label, ask your grocer. If he doesn't know, consider looking elsewhere.

Some grocery chain stores are now labeling fruits and vegetables with their country of origin and indicating whether the produce is traditionally grown (i.e., grown with pesticides and fertilizers) or organic.

Are some fruits and vegetables more likely than others to carry pesticide residues?

Yes. According to the Environmental Working Group (www.ewg.org), which produces an annual "dirty dozen" list of fruits and vegetables containing the highest pesticide residues, the most pesticide-heavy types of produce, as of 2016, were:

Strawberries
Apples
Peaches
Celery
Grapes
Cherries
Spinach
Tomatoes
Sweet bell peppers
Cherry tomatoes
Cucumbers

This makes sense: fruits and vegetables with soft skins and edible outer layers are more likely to deliver pesticides in human consumption than those with removable skins and shells.

Conversely, the EWG's "clean fifteen," the least pesticide-burdened fruits and vegetables are:

Avocados
Sweet corn
Pineapples
Cabbage
Sweet peas
Onions
Asparagus
Mangoes
Papayas
Kiwi
Eggplant

Honeydew melon
Grapefruit
Cantaloupe
Cauliflower

Regardless of which list a food item lands on, it behooves consumers to wash all produce thoroughly before consuming it (particularly greens and anything with a waxy coating).

EWG updates the website (www.ewg.org) frequently with new information on pesticide levels in fruits and vegetables.

Do terms like local and in season really matter when it comes to fruits and vegetables?

Yes. If you can't find organic produce, your next best option is to buy produce that's been grown locally. In general, locally grown fruits and vegetables, raised on small local farms, are not treated with as many chemicals as produce grown far away. That's partly because locally grown produce doesn't need to be picked unripe, then ripened with chemicals, and then treated with preservatives for the long cross-country (or international) trip.

Buying produce that is in season at your location is another way to make sure you're getting fresh, local produce. The reasoning behind this is simple: in-season fruits and vegetables are ample and are found close by during their harvest seasons, and the economics of food favor goods that are close over goods from afar. An internet search for "produce in season now" can be a valuable guide as you search to find the least pesticide-heavy food.

Another tip—get to know local farmers, either through the farmer's market or through the outlet where their produce is sold. Find out which farmers are using organic techniques and working to minimize or eliminate the use of pesticides on their crops. Choose these farmers over those who are using pesticides more heavily. Less pesticide is better; none is best.

Finally, exercising your power as a consumer can have a profound impact on the food that's made available in stores in your region. The simplest and most direct way to influence this is for you, your neighbors, and your friends to communicate directly with your grocer. Some grocery stores now label their produce much more clearly than before. Look for store signs in the produce aisles that tell you whether fruits and vegetables are local or not. In response to consumer demand, some stores give the name of the state or country in which the produce was grown. Others display their certified organic produce on a separate display within the fruit and vegetable section. Encourage whoever sells you your food to do the things you want them to do; it behooves them to listen.

What are food additives, and do they have health consequences?

Food additives is a blanket term that refers to the stabilizers, preservatives, emulsifiers, artificial colors, and flavorings added to foods—fresh and processed—to increase their shelf life. They are the sprays used to make unripe tomatoes red, or to make ground beef look fresher, or the sweetener meant to deliver a certain taste without additional calories.

The evidence base surrounding the safety of these products is woefully small, but this lack of safety testing, these chemicals have been deemed sufficiently safe by the Food and Drug Administration to remain in circulation. This doesn't mean that revelations won't come later; the food industry has been known to recall products found to be unsafe long after they were released to market, and many chemical additives can take years or even decades to manifest harm.

Using the theory of "better safe than sorry" (also called "prudent avoidance"), eating as naturally as possible is the best practice for maintaining a healthy lifestyle. This means minimizing exposure to the things that are thought to be linked to health threats, even though the research on these threats may be incomplete or years away. Use your common sense to determine just how much work you're willing to do to avoid items and lifestyles that may prove hazardous to the health of adults and children.

Even if there are no known adverse health effects from a particular food additive, it's still not a bad idea to limit a child's exposure to it whenever possible. Fresh food without preservatives, processing, and additives is always better than processed foods.

What's the deal with genetically modified (GM) foods?

It's complicated. But here is a quick summary of what the controversy over genetically modified foods is all about.

GM engineering involves reconfiguring the genes in crop plants or adding new genes that have been created in the laboratory.

Scientific modification of plants is not something new. Since time began, nature has been modifying plants and animals through natural evolution, meaning that the plants and animals that adapt best to the changing environment survive and pass their genes on to their offspring. Those that are least fit do not survive. Farmers, too, have been helping nature improve crops for generations by saving the seeds of the best tomatoes and apples to use for next year's crop. This is a kind of genetic selection—the most favorable plants succeed.

Seed companies have been contributing to this genetic strengthening, too. Today's seed catalogs show traditional genetic selection at its finest, promising flowers with bigger blooms, tomatoes that ripen early, and new varieties of old species. Genetic selection has always been cultivated, first by nature and later with help from flower growers and farmers. It's nature at its best.

But here's the problem—today's genetic tinkering is not being undertaken by farmers. It is being driven by chemical (i.e., pesticide) manufacturers and plant geneticists, and it is proceeding on a macro scale. The chemical manufacturers' goal is not to produce a tastier apple, a juicier tomato, or more nourishing corn, but rather to modify food crops, such as corn and soybeans, so that the crops will be resistant to the pesticides that these same companies make. Then, when it comes time to weed vast tracts of planted corn or soybeans, the agrobusiness can spray the pesticide-resistant crops with the chemical company's product to kill the weeds—rather than perform the tedious task of mechanical weeding. The weeds die, the crops live, and the pesticide company makes money. At first glance it appears to be an efficient way to weed a big field.

But wait a minute! Those crops are our food. They go into the cereals, snacks, and processed products that we and our kids eat. Won't crop plants absorb some of the pesticides that are sprayed on them while they're growing—especially if more and stronger pesticides are being used on them? All pesticides and herbicides have potential to be toxic to humans, and especially to children.

And what happens when the "survival of the fittest" kicks in? Won't some weeds figure out how to thwart the herbicides? Will this mean that the industrial farmer has to spray more and stronger herbicides to get the job done?

Despite promises by chemical manufacturers that weeds would not become resistant to Roundup (glyphosate, the herbicide most widely used in the United States on genetically modified food crops), resistant weeds are now rampant. It is reported that weeds resistant to Roundup cover more than 100 million acres across several dozen US states. According to the World Health Organization, Roundup is a probable human carcinogen a chemical judged probably capable of causing cancer in humans. To combat the spread of herbicide-resistant weeds, larger and larger quantities of this probable cancer-causing herbicide are now being used. Use of glyphosate has increased in the United States by 2,500% over the past 25 years.

To combat the problem of glyphosate-resistant weeds, chemical companies are now engineering GM seeds to withstand not only to glyphosate, but also to be resistant to two additional, older herbicides: 2,4 D (a component of the notorious Agent Orange, used during the Vietnam War to defoliate jungles) and dicamba (a pesticide highly toxic to birds and other living things). These highly toxic chemicals are now beginning to be added into the chemical regimen sprayed on fields of corn, soybeans, and other commercial crops. In turn, US residents can expect that measurable levels of these toxic chemicals will carry over into the foods produced from these heavily treated crops—with additional chemicals added to pesticide protocols potentially still to come.

Chemical manufacturers have long portrayed the goal of GM foods as being the provision of more nutritious crops capable of feeding the world. But a 2016 *New York Times* report, "Uncertain Harvest," contested this claim, reporting that GM foods crops have actually failed to increase food production or the robustness of crops being harvested. GMO crops have also failed to reduce pesticide use, amounting to another undelivered promise made by pesticide manufacturers.

In sum, genetically modified foods are not inherently unhealthy in themselves. The problem is the company they keep—the additional layers of pesticides of ever-increasing toxicity—pesticides that farmers and growers are beholden to because their seeds are genetically modified to accommodate them. As this GM-industrial complex continues to proliferate, the world's food supply grows increasingly dependent on GM seeds, which in turn increases dependence on chemical fertilizers and pesticides. These chemicals, as discussed at length, are toxic to humans.

So do I buy GM foods or not?

Corn and soy products constitute a growing share of the food consumed by Americans. More than 90% of corn and soy crops in the United States are grown using GM seeds. These crops use large quantities of pesticides, some of which are probable human carcinogens. Therefore, the healthier choice would be to eat only those foods that are certified GM-free. One more reason to eat organic.

What is processed food, and does it contain toxic chemicals?

Definitions of what constitutes "processed food" vary, but it's generally fair to say that a processed food is food that is packaged in a box, can, or bag prior to its sale to consumers. In other words, processed food is the opposite of fresh food.

The processing of food can involve the introduction of ingredients that are not wholesome—and, in some cases, that are toxic.

Here are some processed foods to watch out for.

Hot dogs, bacon, cold cuts, and other processed meats. Most of these products are cured with nitrates; during the cooking process, nitrates can be converted into nitrites and nitrosamines, which are carcinogenic. Hot dogs or bacon that cooked at high heat is likely to have its nitrates converted to nitrites and nitrosamines, landing them high on the list of foods to avoid giving kids. The highest amount of nitrosamines are found in burnt bacon.

Hot dogs and pressed meats have also been the subjects of multiple major product recalls over past years due to contamination with *Listeria*, a bacterium that can cause pregnant women to miscarry and that can cause serious illness in the elderly, infants, and those with immune deficiencies.

Safer versions of hot dogs, bacon, cold cuts, and other processed meats do exist—look for those that have not been cured with nitrates.

Processed cereals. While the addition of nutrients to cereals can help to ensure that children receive some important vitamins and minerals, most processed cereals contain excess sugar and most are now made with GMO cereal crops—and that means they're being treated with heavy doses of pesticides.

Processed baked goods. In addition to the excess of saturated fats and sugars in these foods, the GMO caution applies to them, too.

What is pasteurization, and does it have anything to do with toxic chemicals in food?

Pasteurization is the process in which a liquid, such as milk or cider, is brought to a high enough temperature to kill germs in the product before it is sold for consumption. The pasteurization of milk is responsible for eliminating tuberculosis and other germs in raw milk. Pasteurization contributed to a great reduction in cases of childhood tuberculosis during the 20th century. Today, it continues to provide benefits in protecting our milk supply.

In recent years, many artisanal cheeses are being made from raw milk. Without the pasteurization process, there is no guarantee that these cheeses are safe and free from tuberculosis or other dangerous, disease-causing germs, such as *Salmonella*, *Campylobacter*, and even more exotic bacteria. There are still potent germs that can be present in unpasteurized milk and cheese and infect children and adults.

Pasteurization is also effective in eliminating dangerous bacteria, such as *E.coli* 0157:H7, in products like apple cider. Why apple cider? Farmers often make their apple cider from apples that are bruised from dropping to the ground at harvest time. If there are also cattle on the farm, their droppings may have contained *E.coli* 0157:H7 and contaminated the dirt around the apple trees. When the apples are crushed during the process of making cider, the *E.coli* 0157:H7 contaminates the cider. If the cider is not pasteurized, it can transmit the bacteria to the child or adult who drinks it.

What's the difference between organic and nonorganic dairy products?

All types of milk and yogurt products provide calcium needed for children's bones and development. Organic milk products reduce a child's exposure to the antibiotics and hormones that are widely used in raising non-organic cows and added by the shovelful to their feed. Antibiotics are used to prevent the livestock from developing infections, but they have been linked with the proliferation of antibiotic-resistant strains of bacteria in both humans and animals.

How do I know which fish is safe to eat?

Fish contain important nutrients, especially omega-3 fatty acids that protect against heart disease, and many healthy fats that contribute to heart and brain health. But, depending on where the fish comes from, it can also contain some dangerous chemical contaminants. If your fish lived in a river that was contaminated by pollutants discharged into the river by a factory, it may have picked up some of these contaminants, especially PCBs and mercury. Here is an overview of these two common contaminants:

PCBs. The biggest concerns about eating fish center on polychlorinated biphenyls (PCBs), which, because of industrial pollution, are now found in some fish. PCBs are manufactured chemicals that were widely used in the production of electrical generators and transformers until their ban in the 1970s and still persist in the environment. They enter the environment when they are discharged into rivers by industries, as well as from accidental leaks and spills. PCBs were widely used in industrial settings because they did not break down easily; that same characteristic, though, is why PCBs now appear in places where they were never used or even spilled. Pristine rivers and the far reaches of the Arctic Circle contain traces of both PCBs and dioxins, which are the toxic chemical contaminants that arise from the burning PCBs.

PCBs have contaminated a number of waterways in the United States, including the Great Lakes and the Hudson River, through industrial runoffs and spills. Tiny fish in the waterways consume PCB-contaminated plants and animals. When the larger fish, crabs, and lobsters consume the smaller fish that have eaten the contaminated plants, the PCBs become part of the larger fishes' bodies; this is known as bioaccumulation of PCBs. The larger fish and shellfish in the waters are more heavily contaminated than the smaller fish because they have consumed substantially more of the PCB-laden fish, whose PCBs then become part of the larger fish's body. Eventually, a fisherman catches the fish, and the fish—along with its body burden of PCBs—becomes part of whoever eats it.

PCB-contaminated fish aren't safe for women of child-bearing age to eat because PCBs can cross the placenta from a pregnant mother to the baby; they are linked with a loss of intelligence and behavior problems in children. Studies of children whose mothers ate PCB-contaminated fish from the Great Lakes have confirmed these problems.

Mercury. Mercury is another contaminant that moves up the food chain (bioaccumulates) in the same way as PCBs. Mercury is becoming a more common pollutant in lakes and streams.

Here are some good suggestions that will help you minimize exposure to contaminants in fish:

If you catch your own fish, know the quality of the water where your fish comes from, and don't exceed the recommended frequency for eating fish from that area. Contact your state or local health department or environmental protection agency for a listing of contaminated fishing areas and guidelines about which fish are safe to eat.

If you buy your fish, know where your fish comes from. Wild fish is usually safer than farmed fish, since the farmed fish may be fed with contaminated smaller fish products. Take the same care with crabs, lobsters, and other shellfish and eels since they can have high levels of PCBs and other contaminants from polluted waterways. Know where they came from and how much is safe to eat.

Young, small fish will have fewer contaminants than larger fish. Avoid eating the skin and the fatty layer of fish, where PCBs accumulate.

Pregnant mothers and those with young children should check USDA listings to help choose fish with lower levels of mercury contamination. Here are the 2014 draft guidelines:

Do not eat these fish—they contain high levels of mercury:
Shark
Swordfish
King Mackerel
Tilefish

Do eat these fish and shellfish that are lower in mercury. (Adults can eat up to 6 oz a week, and children should eat 1 to 3 oz a week.)
Shrimp
Pollock
Salmon
Canned light tuna
Tilapia
Catfish
Cod

Check local advisories about the safety of fish caught by family and friends in your local lakes, rivers, and coastal areas. If no advice is available, eat no more than 6 ounces (one average meal) per week of fish you catch from local waters, but don't consume any other fish during that week.

Does ground beef contain E.coli?

Hamburgers that are still red or even pink in the middle can carry a deadly strain of bacteria, *E.coli* 0157:H7 (one of a class of bacteria called Shiga toxin-producing *Escherichia coli*, or STECs), which has become more common in the cattle industry in the United States and elsewhere. A more virulent strain of the normal *E.coli* bacteria that is found in the digestive tracts of people and animals, *E.coli* 0157:H7 and other STECs cause severe gastrointestinal distress and diarrhea. Children are especially vulnerable to *E.coli* 0157:H7 and can develop life-threatening hemolytic uremic syndrome (HUS) after suffering bouts of bloody diarrhea. More strains of STECs and non-STECs have been developing over the past few years. Recent research published in the journal *Emerging Infectious Diseases* implicates routine antibiotic use in cattle feed as the cause of the propagation of these more virulent bacteria in cattle.

Why are hamburgers more of a problem than meats like grilled steak? That's easy to understand if we look at what happens when cattle carrying *E.coli* 0157:H7 in their digestive system are brought to the slaughterhouse. The bacteria may contaminate the meat in the slaughterhouse or meat-processing plant when fecal material from the cattle comes in contact with the meat. For those cuts of meat that remain intact during processing, such as steaks, the bacterium tends to remain on the outside of the meat. When you grill or sear the meat, the bacteria are killed by the high temperatures, so they are killed when steak is seared or grilled. So, even if you eat your steak rare—visibly pink or red in the center—*E.coli* 0157:H7 may not pose a significant threat because the contamination remained on the outside of the meat and was killed during cooking.

But when hamburger is made, the meat containing the bacteria on the surface is ground up. Any contamination present on the outside of the meat is thoroughly mixed into the center of the meat as well. If you cook the meat to only rare, the bacteria in the center aren't killed and can be passed along to the person who eats the rare hamburger.

Because *E.coli* 0157:H7 can cause severe illness in children (they can die from it), it's extremely important that hamburgers be cooked to an internal temperature of 160°.

Are peanuts toxic for children?

Peanut allergy affects 1.0% to 1.5% of the population. It is not clear why some children develop this life-threatening allergy, but current research suggests that infants who are exposed to peanut butter at an early age are less likely to develop an allergy to peanuts than those who are not exposed to peanuts until they are older. As recommendations have recently been changed, you should carefully discuss this issue with your child's pediatrician prior to introducing peanuts into your child's diet.

The American Academy of Pediatrics makes the following recommendations for parents and pediatrions regarding the introduction of peanuts into the diets of babies:

All babies should be introduced to other solid food before they are offered peanut-containing foods, to be sure they are developmentally ready.

High-risk babies (those with severe eczema and/or egg allergy) should have peanut-containing foods introduced at 4 to 6 months of age only after parental consultation with the baby's pediatrician to determine whether the first taste should take place in a doctor's office or at home under close observation. Allergy testing may be recommended prior to introduction.

Moderate-risk babies (those with mild to moderate eczema) should start peanut-based foods around 6 months at home.

Most babies are low risk, and parents can introduce peanut-based foods along with other solids, usually around 6 months

Building tolerance to peanuts requires making peanut-based foods part of the regular diet, about three times a week.

All parents should discuss these new guidelines with their child's pediatrician during the baby's routine pediatric visit to determine his or her recommendations prior to the introduction of peanuts into the child's diet.

To benefit children in the community with existing life-threatening peanut allergies, many schools have policies on bringing peanut products into school. Some classrooms are "nut free," and some schools do not allow foods containing peanuts to be brought into the school.

A final consideration with peanuts is aflatoxin, a cancer-causing toxin that can develop on moldy peanuts. Commercially processed peanut butter is usually pretty safe from aflatoxin because of the high use of fungicides during the peanut growing season. This is both the good news and the bad news—less aflatoxin, but more pesticide residue. Organic farming doesn't use pesticides, but may have more aflatoxin. To be safe, look for certified organic peanut butter that has been tested for its aflatoxin content. Some of the larger food chains that specialize in organic foods offer this. And be a bit wary about the stores that allow you to make your own peanut butter. If the equipment gets contaminated with aflatoxin from a previous batch of peanuts that had some mold, the peanut butter you grind might pick up aflatoxin, too.

What precautions should be taken to prevent toxic chemicals from getting into a home garden?

Whether it's a few tomato plants on the porch or something much larger, here are a few quick things you should do.

Before planting outdoors, find out the history of the land where you plan to plant. If your neighbors have lived in the area longer than you have, ask them what was there before your house was built. Or check with your local government or health department to be sure your land does not have a questionable environmental history. If your land was previously used for an industrial facility, or a golf course, or a nonorganic orchard, or if it is down hill from and old gas station that may have leaked gasoline from underground storage tanks, your soil may well have toxic material in it.

Choose a spot for your garden that's not close to the edge of the property. If your house is in an older neighborhood, the outskirts of your property may have unwanted chemicals in it. Dumping unwanted chemicals, such as outdated lawn chemicals, automobile oil, and old paints, on the edges of the property was a common practice before the advent of household chemical drop-off sites. Also, if your garden is very close to the property line, any chemicals your neighbor uses may end up in your garden.

Place your garden in a spot that's not too close to a highway or busy street. Runoff from the road can contaminate your garden with chemicals or road salt. Similarly, avoid placing your garden very close to a building that has flaking or chipping paint, which may be old lead paint.

Start a compost pile. A compost pile is a way to turn lawn and vegetable waste into a great fertilizer that will help your garden grow. You might decide to purchase a compost bin the size of an outdoor trash can (available from gardening supply stores or online) or you might want to make a three-stage compost bin where you can pile lawn clippings, vegetable peels, and autumn leaves. There are hundreds of ways to make good compost—some are very easy and some are more time intensive.

Garden organically. When you garden organically, you don't use any synthetic herbicides, fertilizers, or pesticides. Of course, you might think that this would open your garden up to an invasion of insect pests or weeds. But that's not true. You may have a few weeds and some bugs, but there are easy ways to manage them. If you rely on building up the soil quality in your garden with good, rich compost so it's a rich and healthy garden, it will produce a bounty of healthy food.

Choose the least toxic way to edge your garden beds. In the past, many gardeners used pressure-treated lumber to define their garden beds. The advantage of this type of lumber was that it withstands weather and insects better than untreated lumber. But there was a big drawback: old pressure-treated wood was treated with toxic chemicals, such as arsenic, chromated copper arsenate, and others. Studies have shown that these chemicals can leach out of the wood and into the soil— where your hungry garden plants are growing. In all likelihood, the chemicals will find their way into your vegetables. New pressure-treated lumber uses chemicals, too. If you want to frame your garden, use a weather-resistant wood, such as cedar, rather than pressure-treated lumber. Or be creative and make a brick or stone edging.

Feed your compost pile with healthy grass clippings, leaves, and vegetable and fruit peels. The emphasis here is on "healthy"—now that you're not using pesticides, your grass clippings are great. And your leaves are healthy additions to the compost pile, since you're not spraying your trees with pesticides. Your organic vegetable and fruit peels make great compost. Before you know it (i.e., next year), you will have some great soil to add to your garden from your compost pile. Just remember a few points—don't add any animal products, oils, or grease to your compost, and don't add grass clippings if the lawn has been treated with pesticides, herbicides, or other "grow strong and healthy" lawn chemicals. Never put dog waste or cat litter on your compost pile, since dog and cat feces can contain parasites that you don't want in your compost pile or in the food you eat. Then, next planting season, add an inch or two of the healthy, rich, black soil from the bottom of the compost pile to your garden for a bumper crop!

10

TOXIC CHEMICALS AND OTHER HAZARDS IN THE HOME

Each year, poison-control centers across the country receive thousands of calls from frantic parents whose children have accidentally ingested toxic chemicals, prescription drugs, and even toxic houseplants. According to the Centers for Disease Control and Prevention, every day 300 children across the United States are treated in hospital emergency departments for accidental poisonings; of the 300, two children die.

These childhood poisonings are caused by a wide variety of medicines and household chemicals, many of which you undoubtedly have in your house and know are toxic. Safety in the presence of household toxins is all about constructing barriers between them and children—and being aware of other hazards that might not be so obvious.

What is the most effective way to prevent children from ingestion or exposure to toxic chemicals in the household?

In short, lock things up. Lock them with locks. Just putting something "up high" isn't good enough; if there's a way for your kids to get it, they probably will. Locks also need to be age-appropriate. What keeps a 2-year-old child out is not sufficient for a 6-year-old. Of course, although the locks need to be secure enough to thwart your child, they should be easy enough for you to open so that you will actually use them.

Lock up all of the following:

- Prescription and over-the-counter medicines
- Household batteries, especially the newer button-type batteries, which can cause severe gastrointestinal burns if ingested
- Under-sink cabinets
- Laundry detergents and supplies
- Oven and drain cleaners—These are some of the most toxic materials in your home and the best advice is to avoid them completely—See Chapter 6 for safer alternatives
- Basement storage areas/cabinets
- Garage storage areas/cabinets
- Liquor cabinets
- Guns and sporting or self-defense items

Each of the items listed above could come with an exhaustive discussion of individual hazards and dangers. For more detailed information, visit www.ewg.org or www.cdc.gov and read about how most household products can pose a significant threat to children who ingest them or are exposed to them.

Moving day is a very bad day for chemical poisonings. An inordinate number of accidents—including chemical ingestions—occur on days when families are moving. Chemicals are out, visible, and set down in places where they wouldn't be otherwise, and parents have their attention pulled in all directions. On moving day, bad things can be avoided by keeping chemicals locked away, out of sight and reach of children. If something enclosed isn't available, the car trunk can serve as a short-term fix during a move. We suggest you put dangerous and toxic chemicals in a safe place a couple of days before the move to get them out of the way and avoid last-minute regrets.

What is the best thing to do if a child ingests or
is otherwise exposed to a toxic chemical?

Two things to do if you have children – and do them long
before an ingestion happens:

1. Find the phone number of your local poison control
   center and store it in your phone or paste in on your
   refrigerator door.
2. Go to a pharmacy and buy a bottle of syrup of ipecac,
   a medicine induces vomiting when administered, and
   store the ipecac someplace safe (preferably one of the
   places with a lock, as detailed in the previous section).
   Syrup of ipecac is often the first line of defense for a
   child who has been poisoned, but for some poisonings,
   you don't want to induce vomiting. Don't induce vomiting if the substance the child has ingested is caustic
   (such as a drain cleaner or lye) or has an oily petroleum
   or hydrocarbon base (such as paint thinners, furniture
   polish, gasoline, kerosene, or solvents).

**When calling poison control, have the bottle or container
of the product that caused the poisoning in your hand.** Be
prepared to read the product name and number to the poison control or rescue squad staff. You may be told to give the
child syrup of ipecac. Don't give ipecac until you have cleared
it with the poison control center.

**If you're instructed to go to the nearest hospital, bring the
bottle or container of the product that caused the poisoning
with you.** Emergency physicians tell us that when parents
come to the emergency department knowing that their child
has eaten something toxic, only 60% of the time do they know
exactly what their child ate. While doctors can run a toxin panel
(a test to determine what the child has ingested), this isn't an
instantaneous test and it picks up just a few substances. By
the time the results arrive, valuable time has been lost, during
which they could have given the child specific treatments.

How do I safely dispose of unwanted chemicals?

Contact local government or a trash collection service to find out what you should do with such materials. Some communities have established household chemical cleanup days. If your town has one, take advantage of it.

For too many years, the corner of the backyard has been a convenient disposal site for used automobile oil, leftover antifreeze, and the last few ounces of turpentine, gasoline, or herbicide. The storm drain in the street has served as a place to pour detergent solutions used to wash the car, clean the driveway, or wash the house.

At first glance, these seem to be small things. But the amount of materials disposed of in our backyards and in our storm drains add up to major pollution of our soil and waterways. Products like oil, gasoline, and antifreeze contain toxic materials that, disposed of carelessly in the backyard or storm drains, can get into wells, streams, lakes, and groundwater—and end up in our drinking water They can also end up on children when they play outside in contaminated dirt or swim at the local beach.

Your backyard, garage, attic, and basement are no place to discard unwanted chemicals. They shouldn't be put out with regular trash for pickup or thrown in dumpsters, either. Both eventually end up in landfills or are burned in municipal incinerators and come back to us as air, water, or soil pollution that can be damaging to individual and public health. They can also be hazards to trash collectors.

Are all baby products safe and nontoxic?

No. Baby products are all supposed to all be safe, but in reality, some are not. For example, consider products that contain phthalates or bisphenol A (BPA). Knowing what we now know about the toxicity of phthalates and BPA even at very low levels of exposure, parents should take care to avoid these ingredients (and other endocrine disruptors) in the products they choose for a baby. Here are some ideas that should help you.

Baby soap. The best soap for baby is no soap at all—just plain warm water and a washcloth. This should be all you need for swabbing the mild drooling of babies. If your baby is a chronic spitter of milk or formula, use a mild soap, such as an unscented olive-oil castile soap, for cleanups. Once the baby begins to crawl on the floor, the same unscented olive-oil castile soap or unscented, no-additive "baby soaps" are fine to use. Avoid choosing products that have fragrances or additives that make bubbles. Fragrances can cause sensitivities on baby's skin, even when they are "natural." Most manufactured fragrances contain phthalates, which are to be avoided. Soaps that make bubbles are too harsh and may cause urinary tract infections, especially in baby girls.

Baby shampoo. Use fragrance-free baby shampoo—adult shampoos are too harsh for a baby.

Detergents. Make your baby's laundry detergent as mild as possible—no scents, no additives, no color enhancers, no bleaches. Use a detergent specifically designed for infant laundry. Wash your baby's clothes separately from the rest of the family's clothes, as an extra measure of protection for the baby. Your pediatrician will have advice on this topic also.

Diaper rash ointments. Avoid ointments with a long list of ingredients. The more ingredients, the more likely the baby will react to one of them. For preventing and treating diaper rash, choose ointments that are primarily zinc oxide. Plain petroleum jelly is also a good choice for baby's skin.

Wipes. Warm water on a soft cotton pad does the job and protects the baby's skin from the irritation of the alcohol and other ingredients in commercial wipes. A helpful hint is to fill a squirt bottle with warm water and 1 teaspoon of baking soda and use it for quick cleanups. Make new solution every few days.

Is baby powder safe?

No. Baby powder is something to keep out of the baby's room and off the baby. Powder can cause some pretty severe health problems, including pneumonia and lung inflammation when the baby inhales it. Many powders contain particles of talc, a mineral that is a component of talcum powder and that is a close cousin of the dangerous mineral asbestos.

Bottom line—keep all powders, as well as cornstarch (which can cause choking if inhaled by baby) out of the baby's room and breathing range.

Furthermore, talcum powders are not safe for women either. Recent studies are showing that the use of talcum powder in feminine hygiene products can be linked to ovarian cancer. Avoid talcum powder and feminine hygiene sprays, powders, or pads that contain talc.

Are there negative effects of using antibacterial cleaning products?

Yes. At face value, antibacterial cleaners seem like such a good idea. They get rid of germs, and what could be wrong with that?

But think about what you're doing when you kill germs: you kill off the good microbes we all need for survival, along with some of the bad germs. It's important to note the word "some" relative to the bad germs, because antibacterial chemicals don't kill the strongest germs out there. The stronger germs have learned how to get around antibacterial cleaners, so by killing off the competition in the microbe universe (i.e., the weak good germs and the weak bad germs), you now are allowing the stronger germs a free and open playing field to reproduce and to get even stronger.

Our intestinal tracts and digestive systems rely on the good microbes that are stripped away by antibacterial products. It's the same principle that can make prescription antibiotics an unpleasant thing to have to take—often the result is diarrhea or a yeast infection. The way you repopulate your intestine with good microbes is by taking probiotics or eating yogurt. The temporary disruption of the digestive system is not fun.

So what have you accomplished by using antibacterial cleaners? If there were disease-causing bacteria present and they are strong enough to withstand the cleaning agent, you have now enabled stronger, more toxic germs to spread into the area you have just cleaned. Now you and your family will be exposed to a universe of stronger germs, not fewer germs.

Which insect repellants are safe?

Outdoor playtime makes children fair game for mosquito bites. So how can you protect their sensitive skin from bug bites?

For starters, to help minimize the amount of exposed skin, dress your child in lightweight long-sleeved shirts and long pants (when the weather permits). Socks and shoes help prevent the "ankle biters" from getting a chance to bite. Using unscented soaps and shampoos also helps to avoid attracting biting insects.

Beyond that, you may want to consider using insect repellants sparingly, if your child is going to be outdoors for a while in an insect-prone area, or in an area where mosquitoes or other insects are known to be carrying a disease such as dengue fever, Lyme disease, Zika virus, or West Nile virus. Insect repellants should not be used on infants under 2 months of age. Instead, it's best to cover the crib or baby carriage with mosquito netting to protect the infant.

Use an insect repellant that contains either DEET (N,N-diethyl-meta-toluamide) or picaridin (also known as KBR 3023 or icaridin).

Use the lowest strength needed for the job. Read the product label and match the length of exposure time with the strength suggested.

Some "natural" nontoxic insect repellants or skin softeners have been advertised as effective in preventing mosquito bites, such as herb or plant oils. There is little scientific evidence that these products are effective, but some people swear by them.

Is the radiation emitted by mobile phones unhealthy?

Since the advent of mobile phones, consumers and scientists have raised questions about whether electromagnetic radiation (EMF) from the phones is harmful to human health. Evidence from multiple studies globally has been inconclusive, but the studies continue today and prudence is warranted.

As cell phones continue to proliferate and become more available to children and teens, increased exposures to EMFs are occurring. It is known that holding a cell phone to the ear produces measurable absorption of radiofrequency energy in the brain and that children absorb 2 to 10 times as much as adults. A large European study called MOBI-KIDS has been collecting data for several years to determine whether mobile phone use is linked with an increase in brain cancers. Since it is the largest such study done to date, consumers can look forward to the publication of its results in the future.

Meanwhile, you might encourage your child to minimize cell phone use by increasing their use of text messaging (not a difficult sell). The hands-free speakerphone kits that come with most phones keep the phone away from the body, so consider that if you're talking a lot.

What is radon and should I have my home tested for it?

Radon is an invisible gas produced by the radioactive decay of naturally occurring uranium in the earth. In some parts of the country, underground rocks containing uranium produce radon that percolates up through the soil and into the basements of homes, schools, and businesses. In some areas, the levels of radon gas found in homes are high enough to cause health problems. It's estimated that radon gas causes over 10,000 lung cancer deaths annually in the United States.

Because radon is a gas, it seeps readily from the ground into the basements of buildings through cracks in the foundation, in gaps around the household piping, and in well water.

The amount of radon that enters a building depends upon the underlying rock formations in the area and the specific configuration of foundation cracks and air pressure within the house. When radon exists deep in the ground in your area, the intake vents for the hot-air heating system or whole-house roof exhaust fans can draw it into the house. Any situation that causes lower air pressure in the basement than in the outside air can bring radon into the house.

A radon test—either performed by a professional or with a kit purchased at a hardware store—can let you know whether you have radon in your home.

If you decide to do the testing yourself, you'll have two options—a charcoal-based kit or an alpha-detector. A charcoal-based kit is designed for short-term use, and it gives a quick indication of how much radon is accumulating over a few days or a week. An alpha-detector is designed to measure radon over longer periods of time—up to 12 months. Since radon levels in a house can vary over time, this detector generally gives more accurate results than the charcoal-based one, but you have to wait longer for a result.

The bottom line is, if you have over 4 pCi/L of radon in your home, you will want to bring in a trained radon abatement contractor. You can get lists of certified radon inspectors from your state or local health departments or from one of the Environmental Protection Agency's ten regional offices.

A radon abatement contractor may take a variety of measures to correct the radon in your home. The first priority will be to find out how the radon is getting in, so the contractor will check your drains, cracks in the basement walls, and your water supply. (If you have radon in your home and you get your water from a well, make sure you get that tested, too!) Some short-term radon control measures include opening windows, blowing outdoor air into the house with a window fan, and venting crawl spaces. Long-term measures include pumping air into the basement and sealing radon entry routes.

If you're thinking about turning a basement room into living quarters, a den, or a playroom, make sure you have it tested for radon first. If you need to do major renovations, ask your contractor about using techniques to minimize radon levels in the room over the long term. Keep in mind that construction can change radon levels, so retest your house after the construction is completed.

What is asbestos and how do I know if it's in my home?

Asbestos is a white fibrous mineral that was used extensively until the early 1970s in home construction due to its fire-retardant and insulating properties. Very old furnaces and pipes were covered with thick, white, bandage-like asbestos to prevent furnace fires and heat loss. Asbestos is a powerful human carcinogen. All forms of asbestos can cause cancer. Researchers believe that asbestos' carcinogenic properties stem from its fine, fibrous composition—it sheds particles so tiny that humans can inhale them deep into their lungs. Because lungs can't clear the particles, they act as focal spots for cancers to develop. Both lung cancer and mesothelioma, a type of cancer associated almost exclusively with asbestos exposure, can result.

Asbestos has also been used extensively in roofing shingles, floor tiles, and auto brake linings. A form of asbestos called tremolite is found in some brands of play sand, as well. (Check the label on play sand to make sure it does not contain tremolite. If it's not labeled "tremolite-free," don't buy it.)

Evaluation of a home for possible asbestos should be performed by an EPA- certified or state-certified contractor. The contractor should be able to:

Show you his asbestos license or training certificate
Point out areas in your home where he'll need to remove or encapsulate asbestos
Test the questionable material

Provide documentation showing that the asbestos will be taken to an approved landfill or disposal area

Avoid dispersing asbestos fibers outside the work area through encapsulation of the area

Prevent asbestos from getting into the air circulation system of your house.

Is it okay to have exposed fiberglass insulation in the less-inhabited parts of my home?

It's common for contractors or home-construction crews to leave some extra rolls of fiberglass insulation stored in your attic or basement. (It's typically pink or white with brown backing paper.) While the fiberglass looks soft and fluffy, it should be avoided—don't touch it without work gloves and long-sleeved shirts. And don't let children play with it—it's glass, and it can cut, scratch, and irritate skin and lungs!

Since some studies show that fiberglass causes long-term respiratory problems, keep any insulation that hasn't already been installed in a closed plastic bag in your attic or basement so it can't shed tiny particles into the air.

It's also worth noting that if a boat with a fiberglass hull presents the same issues. Make sure that any work done with fiberglass patches is done in a well-ventilated area—preferably outdoors, instead of in a garage or an enclosed area. Respiratory protection should be used, also, if the patches need to be sanded.

Are houseplants toxic?

Some of the most beautiful houseplants are actually quite toxic to children, and many plants should be off limits for pets. (Check the ASPCA website for pet information.) It may be wise to give away plants that appear on the wrong side of Table 10-1.

Table 10-1 Some Toxic and Safer Houseplants

Some Toxic Houseplants		Some Safer Houseplants	
Botanical Name	Common Name	Botanical Name	Common Name
Alocasia spp.	Elephant's ears	*Saintpaulia ionantha*	African violet
Aloe vera	Aloe	*Pilea* spp.	Aluminum plant
Amaryllis spp.	Amaryllis	*Nephrolepis exaltata*	Boston fern
Caladium spp.	Angel wings	*Schlumbergera bridgesii*	Christmas cactus
Chrysanthemum spp.	Chrysanthemums	*Coleus hybridus*	Coleus
Cyclamen spp.	Cyclamen	*Crassula argenta*	Jade plant
Dieffenbachia spp.	Dumb cane	*Kalanchoe* spp.	Kalanchoe
Epipremnum aureum	Golden pothos	*Plectranthus* spp.	Swedish ivy
Philodendron spp.	Philodendrons	*Aphelandra squarrosa*	Zebra plant

Remember that individual sensitivities are different—what doesn't bother one person might cause sensitivity in another. That said, you might want to try some of the safer house plants, if you want to brighten up a corner.

11

DAYCARE

Finding the right caregiver for a child outside of home can be a challenge—financially, logistically, emotionally. An added concern, and surely one on most parents' minds when touring a prospective childcare facility, is whether the environment and facilities are safe, healthy, and clean. So no matter what sort of care you choose—whether it's leaving your child in the home of a family member or enrolling the child at a licensed daycare—this chapter gives a list of questions to ask (along with criteria for the responses) to make sure your child is safe from environmental hazards in the daycare setting. (Although this chapter is on topics specific to daycare, things covered elsewhere in the book may be helpful, too.)

Does the daycare facility meet fire-safety codes?

Fire safety for licensed daycare facilities is regulated by law. The law requires that nonflammable construction materials be used, that emergency exits be available, that smoke and possibly carbon monoxide alarms be installed, and that each staff member be properly trained for a fire emergency. Having your child stay in a building subject to fire-safety regulations is a benefit because the regulations add a measure of protection your child may not get in an unlicensed facility. People who die in fires usually don't die from the fire itself, but from inhaling fumes produced by burning toxic materials. So if your daycare facility meets fire codes, your child is less likely to be exposed to the life-threatening toxic products that result from a fire.

Depending on where you live, many agencies may be involved in regulating licensed daycare, such as the state department of social services or the education department. You should ask the daycare provider:

- When the facility was last inspected by the fire department
- If you can see the results of the inspections done by various agencies
- If the renewal of the permit requires a visit from the fire department or is just a paper submission

Also keep an eye out for warning signs, such as any of the following:

Extension cords. Look for fraying, too many things plugged into the same outlet, or cords strung around the room. Too many cords may indicate an outdated electrical system that can become overloaded and cause a fire.

Gasoline or kerosene room heaters. These heaters are highly flammable. In addition, their vapors can accumulate in confined areas and ignite with explosive results. If the heaters tip over and spill fuel, there could be a fire or an explosion. Because gasoline and kerosene room heaters are so dangerous, they shouldn't be used.

Improper indoor storage. Be on the alert for piles of newspapers, flammable materials stored indoors, and propane tanks or gasoline kept inside the house (which is extremely dangerous).

Smoke hazards. Ask if the chimney, furnace, and water heater are cleaned on a regular basis. Find out about cigarette smoking as well. Do caregivers smoke indoors? Are burning cigarettes ever left unattended? (Remember, no child should be exposed to tobacco smoke.)

Does the daycare facility meet health codes?

Ask your local health department for guidance on how to be sure that a daycare facility is protected against health risks. Some possible environmental hazards you'll want to check for include lead paint (indoors and out) and pesticide use.

Sanitation is another area you'll want to investigate, because children can spread germs through poor sanitation. Make sure all of the toilets work and that there aren't any problems with the septic system. Look in each bathroom to see that it's clean and that there is soap available for hand washing. And, of course, make sure the facility emphasizes the need for every staff member to wash hands after using the bathroom.

Does the daycare facility have a lead problem?

Lead poisoning is a danger to children, especially children under 6 years of age, whose brains and nervous systems are developing. That's why it's really important that the daycare facility doesn't have lead paint.

Lead paint was widely used in buildings built before 1978, and it's safe to assume that any paint applied before 1978 contains lead. Use the same guidelines recommended for your home to be sure the daycare facility is not a source of lead poisoning for your child (see Chapter 5 for a lot more on the topic of lead). Remember, Grandma's house is as likely to have lead paint as any other type of daycare facility if it was built before 1978. You may have lived in the house as a child and had no problems. But, like you, the lead paint in your childhood home is much older now, and the paint may be chipping in places that only a child can find. Take this issue seriously and figure out how you can make Grandma's house safe, if your child is going to be spending time there.

Does the daycare provider lock up all medications?

Most parents have at some point sent their child to daycare with a prescribed medication that needs to be taken while the child is in the daycare facility. And caregivers are just as likely to have a medication with them in their purse or pocket. Make sure that the daycare provider ensures that all medications are locked away from little hands' reach.

Does the daycare provider use nontoxic cleaning products?

Many common household cleaners contain toxic ingredients that children shouldn't be exposed to. After these cleaners are used, traces of them can remain on tabletops, carpets, floors, and toys. And when children crawl on the floor or put toys in their mouths, they may ingest traces of the cleaner. When the cleaners are used properly, exposure to their residues is a minimal risk. Still, accidental ingestion of some of the products can be life-threatening.

Does the daycare provider have a strict hand-washing policy?

Hand washing by both children and caregivers is vital in preventing kids from ingesting toxic materials, such as lead dust or contaminated soil, and in decreasing the spread of communicable diseases.

Daycare workers should wash their hands
- **After using cleaners or products containing chemicals**
- **Before preparing food**
- **After changing a diaper**
- **After wiping a runny nose or cleaning up other infectious materials**
- **After using the toilet**

Children need to wash their hands, too, and you should ask caregivers when they require children to do so. Hand washing after playing outside, after using the toilet, before eating, and after playing with any pets that are kept at the facility is optimal.

Does the daycare use lead-free and asbestos-free crayons?

The possibility of asbestos in crayons is another cause for concern. As recently as 2015, the Environmental Working Group (www.ewg.org) found evidence of asbestos in several toys manufactured in China, including crayons and amateur crime lab kits. The asbestos probably came from talc, a mineral used as a binding agent in crayons and in the loose powder of the "fingerprint kits." Since both the asbestos and talc minerals can be found in the same mines, asbestos is often a contaminant of talc.

Since the Consumer Product Safety Commission does not specifically test for asbestos in crayons, it's best to buy crayons manufactured in the United States by a company that no longer uses talc. Parents can get further information on product research and guidelines from EWG's outreach and education program, Healthy Child–Healthy World, at www.healthychild.org.

The danger of asbestos is most serious if asbestos fibers are inhaled, beginning a cycle of lung scarring that can ultimately lead to asbestos-related diseases, such as lung cancer, in later life. The ingestion of asbestos fibers is also suspected to be related to an increase in cancer of the intestinal tract.

If you are concerned that your child may have been using crayons that had lead or asbestos in them, you don't need to panic. On your next routine visit to the pediatrician, voice your concerns and ask whether your child needs to be tested for lead poisoning. It's an easy screening procedure that's recommended as part of routine pediatric care for children who may have been exposed to lead and involves taking only a few drops of blood from your child's fingertip. As far as asbestos goes, the likelihood that your child could have inhaled enough asbestos to cause health problems later in life just from using crayons is very small. In fact, there are no blood tests or other screening tests that would be helpful at this time. Also, screening a child for asbestos exposure by doing a chest X-ray has no value whatsoever and is strongly discouraged. So the best thing you can do is to make sure your child uses asbestos-free crayons in the future—and then not worry about it.

Keep in mind that a brief exposure to crayons that have asbestos or lead in them is a minimal risk to your child's health, but one you will want to avoid. With asbestos, the risk of disease is also related to other lifestyle risks—for example, someone who smokes is 50 times as likely to develop lung cancer from an asbestos exposure than someone who doesn't smoke. With lead, the child's danger of lead poisoning is dependent upon his total ingestion of lead from a number of different sources. To protect your child from lead poisoning, eliminate every lead source that you can.

Does the daycare provider apply pesticides anywhere in the facility?

Pesticides contain all sorts of toxic chemicals that may be harmful to children. For that reason, kids shouldn't be exposed to pesticides at all.

Also ask your daycare to be aware of any pesticide spraying going on in the neighborhood, so that the children are not playing outdoors while pesticide is being sprayed next door. A number of states or municipalities have dealt with this issue by enacting "neighbor notification" laws for commercial pesticide spraying. Under such laws, neighbors must receive advance warning (usually 24 hours) of pesticide spraying that will be done on adjacent properties. This gives parents or daycare staff enough time to cover the outdoor toys or to bring them inside, to close the windows, and to keep children indoors while pesticide is being sprayed next door.

Does the play area contain toxic materials or pressure-treated lumber?

You probably expect an outdoor play area to have swings, slide, sandboxes, jungle gyms, and the like. What you shouldn't expect to see anywhere near the play area, however, are cans of weed killer, pesticides, spray paint, turpentine, lawn mower oil, gasoline, and cleaning materials. Toxic products either should not be used at all, or at the very least, should be locked away in an area that's not accessible to children.

Don't overlook old playground equipment made from pressure-treated lumber. Before being phased out in 2003 because of concerns about its health hazards, pressure-treated lumber used for decks, picnic tables, and even children's play structures contained arsenic. To make lumber more weather-proof, a chemical called chromated copper arsenate (CCA) was used to soak the wood under pressure. Most of us have seen the green-tinged, damp look of pressure-treated wood.

In 2003, the Environmental Working Group (www.ewg.org) did some sampling of the soil around pressure-treated wood decks and playground equipment and found elevated levels of arsenic in the soil. It was clear that the arsenic had leached out of the pressure-treated wood into the dirt where children play. EWG did some projections of how long it would take before the wood would stop releasing the arsenic and the results were not encouraging. Their data indicated that arsenic would probably leach out of the pressure-treated wood for many years.

If your daycare center has picnic tables, playscapes, or decks made from old pressure-treated lumber that have not been replaced by safer products, parents should insist on the following precautions.

- Sandboxes or similar play spaces should not be located under old pressure-treated decking or within old pressure-treated play structures.
- If children are allowed to play on old pressure-treated play structures at the daycare, daycare workers should supervise careful hand washing after playtime and before eating.
- Table coverings should be used on pressure-treated wood picnic tables where the child has snacks or lunch, to prevent foods from resting directly on the wood.

12

SCHOOLS

School is a time for new experiences for both parent and child. New learning situations challenge and help the child grow to meet ever larger challenges in the world. But the school environment may contain exposures to environmental hazards that can detract from the child's ability to grow and thrive. This chapter details both the most common hazards and attainable parental interventions for the school environment.

How can I find out if my child's school has had lead or asbestos problems in the past?

The Parent-Teacher Association (PTA), principal, and school custodian are the best parties to reach out to. Here are the questions to ask:

- How old is the school building? If it was built before 1978, has anyone evaluated whether there is lead paint inside or outside?
- If the school was built before 1978, has the school been painted recently? If so, who did it? Was the outside of the school sandblasted? Did anyone check to see if there was lead paint on the school before the sandblasting was done?
- If the school was built before 1978, have renovations been done to the school's interior? If so, was it evaluated

by a certified lead paint contractor before renovations were started? Was there lead paint in the school? Was it properly removed by a certified lead paint abatement contractor?

- Has any part of the school been demolished to make way for new construction? Was it evaluated for lead paint and asbestos prior to demolition? If either lead paint or asbestos were present, were they removed in accordance with appropriate guidelines? How was the rest of the school protected from the dust caused by the demolition?
- Have the school's drinking water and fountains been tested for lead?
- Has there been any recent construction in the school?
- How has the school's boiler or furnace been working? Was there ever asbestos in the area of the school's furnace?
- Has a new furnace been installed? If so, how recently was this done? What happened to the old furnace? What happened to the asbestos covering the old furnace or the heating pipes that carry heat to the other parts of the building? Was is removed or abated in place? Is there still asbestos in the school? Where?
- Have the ceiling tiles throughout the school been evaluated by a certified asbestos abatement professional? Do any of them have asbestos? What recommendations have been made regarding their replacement or maintenance?
- Have the athletic fields been sprayed with pesticides or replaced with artificial turf? Are the least toxic materials being used?

Once you find out the answers to these questions, you will have a better idea whether there is a potential problem and a hint at its severity. This information should help you determine what should happen next. (Refer to Chapter 5 for more background on the topics listed above.)

What are the implications and complications of lead in school buildings?

If you've been reading this book in sequential order, you know by now how serious the threat of lead poisoning is to your child's health. Chipping, peeling, and flaking lead paint is an especially serious health hazard for children under the age of 6 years. If your school has a nursery, kindergarten, or daycare, they are the most vulnerable areas—and the places you want to focus on in your discussions of lead paint in schools. If these classrooms haven't already been checked for lead paint, they definitely should be. If lead paint is present, call your local or state health department to find out what steps need to be taken to ensure that the children are not at risk for lead poisoning.

Another potentially serious source of lead poisoning in schools is caused by untrained workers who sandblast lead paint on the outside of the school building or an adjacent building, or who use a propane torch to remove old lead paint from interior or exterior trim. Power-sanding lead paint can create a lot of airborne lead dust and can also result in accumulation of leaded debris inside and outside the school. Torching lead paint can create highly toxic lead fumes that children, teachers, and workers can inhale.

If you discover that workers have power-sanded lead paint at your school or an adjacent building or that uncertified contractors have done renovations in areas where lead paint is present, contact your local or state health department immediately for guidance on what you need to do. You may need to have the school get the dust tested to determine whether elevated lead levels are present. You may want to bring the issue to the attention of the school's PTA or their environmental committee. Their next step may be to ask that the school call in a certified lead paint removal contractor for a professional assessment and cleanup so that the school will be safe for your children. Children exposed to lead dust may need to be screened by their pediatrician (a simple blood lead test should do it), to make sure they do not have elevated blood lead levels.

What are the implications of asbestos being present in a school building?

Asbestos is an umbrella term for a group of six naturally occurring fibrous minerals. Asbestos mines in Canada, Russia, Brazil, and South Africa produce rocks containing thin, nearly indestructible asbestos fibers that resist heat, acid, and fire. Since the 1920s, billions of tons of asbestos have been used in homes, schools, and public buildings. The heaviest use of asbestos occurred in buildings built in the 1950s and 1960s. In the 1970s, the use of asbestos rapidly declined as the health hazards of asbestos became better known. These hazards include lung cancer and malignant mesothelioma (a cancer of the chest and abdominal lining). These cancers can occur years after a person inhales asbestos fibers. Lung cancer can occur 10 to 30 years after exposure to asbestos fibers, while mesothelioma generally occurs 20 to 50 years after exposure. All new use of asbestos in all forms is now banned in the United States.

If you suspect your school contains asbestos, work through the PTO or PTA to ask the school to arrange for a certified inspector to perform a visual inspection, if this has not been done in the past. The inspector will examine pieces of suspect material under an electron microscope to determine whether the material is really asbestos. It is not helpful for the inspector to take an air sample. Air sampling identifies only the asbestos particles that are airborne at a single moment in time, and asbestos is released into the air intermittently, such as when a hot-air heating system comes on and blows particles throughout the building, or when the asbestos is disturbed in some way—by a leak, or a breeze, or activities in the area.

Should asbestos be removed from a school building?

Although the hazards of asbestos and the dangers of improper asbestos removal were known by the 1970s, asbestos-related incidents occurred some 20 years later in schools in New York City and in New Jersey in the early 1990s. Old asbestos that had been applied as ceiling insulation and placed in ceiling tiles deteriorated in these schools over the summer and white asbestos particles that looked like snow were present on the children's desks when they came back to school in September. By that time, the federal Asbestos Hazard Emergency Response Act (AHERA) law was in place and schools were inspecting and removing asbestos as required by law. Unfortunately, in New York City, unqualified asbestos contractors were hired to do some of the asbestos removal and they created asbestos contamination throughout the city.

Parental concerns reached a fever pitch. Debate raged over what should be done, and the opening of schools was delayed. As a result of the very public discussion about the problem, health and municipal officials developed guidelines about when asbestos should be removed from buildings and when it's safer to encapsulate it and leave it in place. These guidelines are solid and well thought through. Here they are:

- If asbestos is in poor condition, with apparent flaking and friability, it needs to be removed immediately by a licensed, certified asbestos removal expert. This work needs to be done when children are away from the school.
- If the asbestos is in good condition, with no flaking or cracking, it's better to leave well enough alone, to create a written record of its presence, to consider putting physical barriers between it and children, and to continue to monitor its condition on a regular basis.

What if my child has already been exposed to asbestos in his school?

If your child has already been exposed to asbestos, don't panic. He doesn't need to have any sort of medical screening, because asbestos exposure doesn't produce any detectable physical damage until an average of 20 to 50 years after exposure. In particular, don't get a chest X-ray. It will reveal nothing in regard to the asbestos and will only expose your child to unnecessary radiation. Instead of worrying, use all your parental insights, guidance, and teaching to make sure your child does not become a smoker. People exposed to asbestos and who take up smoking are 50 times more likely to develop asbestos-related lung cancer than people exposed to asbestos who don't smoke.

So don't wait until your child is a teenager to talk about smoking. These days, smoking is a childhood disease. According to national statistics, the vast majority of adult smokers began smoking in their childhood or teens. Few adults take up smoking. So begin to have those conversations when your child is 7 or 8 years old.

What can parents do to demand action or transparency related to asbestos?

The 1984 federal Asbestos Hazard Emergency Response Act (AHERA) was passed to protect children and school employees from the hazards of asbestos in the schools. Federal funds were made available to financially needy schools for investigation and remediation.

Under AHERA, schools are required to systematically inspect every room and every surface for the presence of asbestos every 3 years and to keep a written record of the findings. The inspections must be done by properly qualified professional inspectors, and parents and teachers must be informed of the inspections.

You can make sure that the legally mandated inspections under AHERA were done in your child's school. Under federal law, parents have the right to request and examine the school's asbestos records. If the school administration doesn't respond to a written request for records, report it to the nearest Environmental Protection Agency (EPA) regional office.

Make sure that proper asbestos abatement was done if asbestos was found. A review of school records should show whether a properly trained asbestos contractor did the work.

An asbestos problem that has been taken care of by a certified asbestos abatement contractor should leave you with nothing to worry about. But if, instead, inexperienced and uncertified contractors did the abatement, immediately contact EPA and your local or state health department for guidance on what to do.

How can I make sure that the drinking water in my child's school is lead-free?

In many older schools, the drinking water is contaminated by lead because some older schools, like older homes, have lead pipes in their plumbing. They may also have lead solder in their plumbing (lead solder was not banned from use by the federal government until 1986). When water sits in lead pipes overnight, over a weekend, or during school vacations, a small quantity of lead from the plumbing system can dissolve ("leach") into the drinking water. This is particularly likely to happen in areas where the water is acidic. The recent outbreak of lead poisoning in the whole community of Flint, Michigan, attests to the danger of improperly managed drinking water.

Lead has also been found in some types of school water fountains. When children drink water from these fountains, they will also ingest the lead that is present in the water. Since childhood lead poisoning results from a child's cumulative exposure to lead from many sources in the environment—such as ingesting lead paint chips and dust, along with lead in drinking water—it's important to eliminate lead from every possible source.

The EPA is concerned about lead in drinking water in schools and has published guidelines for schools to prevent lead poisoning. Under the guidelines, schools are required to test their water in a prescribed fashion. If lead is detected in the water, the source must be identified and the problem must be fixed.

What precautions should be in place for a school science lab?

New science and chemistry laboratories use far fewer toxic materials than older chemistry laboratories. The National Institute for Occupational Safety and Health publishes a set of guidelines for chemistry laboratories in schools (NIOSH Publication No. 2007-107). The American Chemical Society has produced a guide, "Reducing Risks to Students and Educators from Hazardous Chemicals in a Secondary School Chemical Inventory," to provide appropriate guidance for chemicals used in secondary school chemistry labs. Well-managed science experiments should pose no threat to a child's health.

However, what may be sitting on the shelf in the old science lab storage closet can yield a frightening array of toxic and even explosive materials, some of which pose life-threatening hazards. Some materials that have been found in high school chemistry labs' old storage areas are included in Table 12-1.

Given the number of chemicals that can cause serious problems in a science class, as a parent working with the PTA (or their environmental committee) in or near a high school with a chemistry lab, you should:

- Ask the school administration for permission to review their protocol and procedures for maintenance of the chemistry storage room.
- Find out how old the school is and how long chemicals have been stored there.
- Determine when the storeroom was last surveyed for aging chemicals and by whom.
- Ask what teachers do to be sure they don't have old or unlabeled chemicals on their shelves.
- Find out if there are any other old storage areas where school chemicals are kept.

If your school doesn't have any sort of protocol for maintaining science lab chemicals, contact your local health department

Table 12-1 Old chemicals potentially in storage

Chemical	Hazard
Benzene	A highly toxic solvent that can cause leukemia.
Carbon tetrachloride	A versatile and universal solvent that was once so widely available that it was used in hobby stamp collecting to bring out the water marks on the stamps. It's highly toxic to the liver and shouldn't be used without respiratory and skin protection.
Ether	Highly explosive. As ether ages, it can form explosive peroxides. Removal of old containers of ether requires a bomb squad.
Hexane	Acute inhalation exposure causes dizziness, giddiness, slight nausea, and headache. Chronic exposure causes nervous system dysfunction, numbness of the extremities, muscular weakness, blurred vision, headache, and fatigue.
Old hydrochloric acid (HCl) or sulfuric acid (H_2SO_4)	Deteriorating containers of hydrochloric acid or sulfuric acid can emit toxic fumes that can react with other lab chemicals. The acids can cause burned lungs if inhaled.
Old hydrofluoric acid	Hydrofluoric acid is a highly toxic substance that can eat through bone and etch glass. It shouldn't be used in high school laboratories. If hydrofluoric acid is in a deteriorating container, it poses a direct health threat to anyone who touches it.
Mercury	Elemental mercury vaporizes readily at room temperature and is extremely toxic if inhaled or handled. It causes brain damage.
Picric acid	Aging picric acid can crystallize and can explode when jostled or even moved on the shelf. Removal requires a bomb squad.
Toluene	Toluene is a toxic solvent; breathing high levels of toluene affects brain function and can cause central nervous system symptoms, such as headaches, confusion, dizziness, sleepiness, and memory loss.

or fire department and ask whether they routinely inspect school laboratory storage rooms. If not, ask if they know who is responsible for doing so.

What precautions should be in place for art studios?

Art supplies can contain lots of toxic substances.

How can you make sure that all the art products in your child's school are safe to use? The good news is that, in 1998, the federal government passed the Hazardous Art Materials Act. Crayons, paint sets, chalk, modeling clay, colored pencils, and other art products must be labeled to show whether the materials contain the potential to cause a chronic hazard. If the materials are not toxic, the label will state "Conforms to ASTM D-4236."

A good project for the PTA environmental committee would be to review the art supplies used by the art class and to recommend that the least-toxic alternatives be used whenever possible. The discussion below covers a list of art supplies and the toxic materials that may be in them.

Oil paints. Oil paints aren't for children. If older teens are interested in taking up oil painting, art teachers need to ensure that safe methods of handling oil paints are taught. Only serious students of art who are willing to take the extra care needed to prevent toxic exposures should be allowed to use oil paints.

Among other things, the art teacher should make sure that budding artists never put the tips of brushes in their mouths. This ancient, very dangerous method of "tipping the brush" has been used by artists to bring the fine hairs of the brushes together to ensure a fine line. The problem is that any brush used for oil painting is likely to have traces of highly toxic metals in it, even if it is cleaned according to directions.

The beautiful colors of cadmium yellow, cobalt blue, manganese blue, and cadmium orange are but a few of the oil paints that contain very toxic metals. And although lead is now prohibited in household paint, lead paint is still available to artists. Some white paints, such as "cremintz white" and "flake white," are mostly lead. It's fairly easy to confirm this—an oil paint that is mostly lead is considerably heavier than an equivalent size tube of another oil paint. Art students must also be cautioned not to sand "high spots" of paint that have accidentally accumulated thicker than desired and dried on their work—even light sanding will release toxic metals into the environment and toxic dust can get onto fingers and be ingested. A better way to handle the problem is to examine the canvas before leaving it to dry overnight. Remove an undesired accumulation of paint while it is wet, with a palette knife. Art teachers often suggest that students "soften the edges" before leaving the paint to dry. This is easily accomplished with a light touch with a soft brush and helps avoid the accumulation of too much paint where you don't want it.

When using solvents to clean brushes, students should use turpenoid or another low-volatility, safer solvent, rather than turpentine. The art classroom should also be adequately ventilated and should not smell of accumulated solvents.

Pastels. Because imported pastels can contain toxic heavy metals, such as lead, cadmium, and mercury compounds, art students should be careful not to inhale the dust. Pastels are not good art supplies for children. Although oil pastels are not as dusty as chalk pastels, they may still contain toxic heavy metals if the pastels are imported. Use ASTM D-4236-approved chalk instead.

Markers. Make sure the markers do not contain toxic solvents and are ASTM D-4236 approved. Avoid scented markers, which can encourage children to taste them. And be aware that most scents that are used in commercial products contain phthalates, an endocrine-disrupting chemical.

Rubber Cement. Rubber cement contains n-heptane, a solvent that can cause dizziness, headache, and unconsciousness at higher doses. Substitute water-based glue, such as white glues, or double-sided tape.

Spray Adhesives. Avoid spray-on adhesives. They contain petroleum distillates and a variety of other chemicals, such as propane, acetone, and isopropyl alcohol. Exposure to the substances through inhalation can cause dizziness, headaches, drowsiness, lack of coordination, and other symptoms. Sometimes people can even "taste" the solvents, many minutes after the aerosol spray has stopped. This is not something you want your child exposed to.

If use of a spray adhesive is a critical requirement for a specific art project by an older student pursuing serious art studies, the student should make sure it is used in a well-ventilated space (like outdoors), with appropriate OSHA (Occupational Safety and Health Administration)-approved respiratory protection. Or the student can choose a CP/AP clear acrylic emulsion to fix the project. (CP/AP stands for Certified Product/ Approved Product. For a product to carry either of these seals, an authority on toxicology from an art and craft materials institute must have evaluated the product and determined that there aren't materials in sufficient quantity to be toxic or to injure the body, even if ingested.)

Pottery and Ceramics. Children who do pottery or ceramics must be old enough to keep their hands out of their mouths when working with pottery and ceramics. The teacher should minimize dust by appropriate methods, and the class should use only nontoxic, certified lead-free paints and glazes.

What is a hazardous spill plan and do schools need them?

Occasionally, schools experience spills that can be hazardous to children's health, such as oil tank overflows or spills of cleaning materials. Many times these spills are not part of a school's emergency plan. Valuable time is wasted while someone waits for staff to figure out which agency is responsible for helping them with the problem.

So check your school's protocol for the handling of spills. If it doesn't have one, offer to write one. Then do some research on protocols that other schools have used. Some potential spills you will want to cover in your protocol are:

- Science lab accidents, including a broken mercury thermometer
- Oil tank overfills and other petroleum spills
- Sewage spills or sewage malfunctions
- Spills of the cleaning agents used in the school

You'll also want to include protocols for the accidental mixing of different cleaning agents that result in toxic emissions (such as mixing of bleach and ammonia-based cleaning agents). And don't forget a protocol for dealing with over-application of pesticides in the classroom, food-service area, or sports field.

A good protocol should list who is in charge, along with two backup contacts. The phone numbers (day, evening, and weekend) should be listed for all of the people in charge. The phone numbers should also be registered with the local police and fire departments.

The protocol should spell out in detail what has to happen, step by step, for any situation—and any others that may be identified as potential problems in the area of your school (such as a spill at an industrial site in the neighborhood).

Ask the school to submit your protocol to the appropriate agency for review and comment; once it is approved, ask the school to adopt it as an official protocol of the school.

Is artificial turf safe?

It depends on the type of turf. In the past decade, manufacturers of artificial turf have aggressively marketed their products to local school boards and athletic boosters. They claim that artificial turf is more durable than natural grass, which can wear down over a long season and collect puddles after a rain.

But artificial turf can have several problems, depending on the materials used to produce it. The most dangerous form of synthetic turf is made from shredded, recycled car and truck tires. This turf poses several hazards:

- **Heat**. On hot summer days with the sun beating down, the temperatures on fields made of shredded tires have reached 140° Fahrenheit. These high temperatures are extremely dangerous, especially for young children playing on the fields at full speed. Dehydration and heat stroke can result.
- **Toxic chemicals**. 1,3-Butadiene, a major chemical component of car and truck tires, is a known human carcinogen—cancer-causing chemical. Old tires can also pick up lead and other hazardous materials during their months and years of running down the road.

The safest course is to put in a natural grass field that is properly drained to prevent puddles and that is seeded with varieties of grass that are tough enough to withstand a sports season. Companies have now emerged that specialize in construction of such fields. Another option is to go with a synthetic turf field made of a material that has been tested and proven safer than old tires.

Can school buildings be worked on structurally (i.e., roof repair) while school is in session?

Roofing tars contain noxious and hazardous materials derived from petroleum products (polycyclic aromatic hydrocarbons). Research has shown that workers who use roofing tars and pitches on a regular basis have as much as 5 times greater risk of lung cancer than the rest of the population.

When roofing tars and pitches are heated, they emit noxious fumes that can cause eye and nose irritation, nausea, headaches, and malaise. That's why the ideal situation involves doing any roofing repairs when the school is not in session. If roofing projects for your school must take place during the school season, recommend that the school administration ensure that the contractors:

- Turn off air intakes in the vicinity while applying tars.
- Close windows on the side of the building where roofing vapors are present.
- Keep the pot of roofing tar away from the area where fumes will get into classrooms. They should also keep the pot covered when they're not using it.

EPILOGUE

Are children adequately protected from environmental toxins today?

The answer to this question is unequivocally "no." Despite a rapidly growing body of medical research showing the effects of toxic chemicals on children's health, and despite decades of work to pass legislation to protect children from environmental toxins, children are still exposed every day to harmful chemicals—in household products, in foods, in the air, in the water. Many of these chemicals have never been tested for safety or toxicity. They therefore pose a clear and present danger to children—a danger that has too long been overlooked by our nation's leaders and continues to be overlooked today.

The clock is ticking as another generation of children is exposed to toxic chemicals in the environment. These chemicals can damage children's developing brains, lungs, reproductive organs, and immune systems, and the chemicals' effects may last throughout children's lifetimes—even into the lives of their children.

The urgency of this threat has not been lost on governments outside the United States. The European Union has recognized the dangers of environmental hazards, and despite strong and continuing opposition from the chemical industry, has developed strong policies to reduce exposures to toxic chemicals among children in Europe. In the US, legislative efforts to stem the flow of untested chemicals into the environment (or even to pay for the clean-up of existing chemical wastes) have been slow to arrive and are lobbied against at every turn by the chemical industry. So long as the uncontrolled flow of corporate money into political campaigns is allowed to continue, toxic environmental exposures will likely persist.

As this book goes to print, the US Environmental Protection Agency is undergoing budgetary and program cuts unlike any in its history; hundreds of hard-won protections against air and water pollution are being thrown out. Toxic pesticides known to damage children's brains are being allowed to stay on the market. Enforcement of the 2016 Lautenberg Safe Chemicals Act appears to be at a standstill. Scientists who have spent their lives working within EPA to protect the environment and human health are being forced out. The protection of children is taking a back seat to the profits of multinational chemical corporations.

The final five chapters of this book provide families and parents with individual solutions that offer a degree of control over the problem of toxic chemical exposures within homes, schools, and communities. These practical steps—large and small—are very important and proven effective. The safe removal of lead-based paint and asbestos from homes will prevent lead poisoning and cancer; eating organic fruits and vegetables reduces pesticide exposure by 90% and improves children's health; cleaning up mold reduces asthma; buying an organic mattress reduces a child's exposure to brain-damaging chemical flame retardants. All of these actions will improve a child's health.

But important as these steps are, our society cannot shop or clean its way out of the problem of toxic chemical exposure. Any consequential change in this space will require collective action, specifically the involvement of parents, legislators, and advocates to assure the security of the environment for future generations. That, perhaps, will be the next book that someone writes.

RESOURCES AND REFERENCES

General References on Children's Health, Toxic Chemicals, and the Environment

Links

Centers for Disease Control and Prevention	www.cdc.gov
Environmental Working Group	www.ewg.org
International Agency for Research on Cancer	www.iarc.fr
National Cancer Institute	www.cancer.gov
National Institutes of Environmental Health Sciences	www.niehs.nih.gov
Natural Resources Defense Council	www.nrdc.org
Environmental Protection Agency	www.epa.gov
US National Library of Medicine, MedlinePlus	www.medlineplus.gov

Table R-1 Regional offices of the US Environmental Protection Agency

Region 1 (CT, MA, ME, NH, RI, VT)
Environmental Protection Agency
5 Post Office Square—Suite 100
Boston, MA 02109-3912
Phone: (617) 918-1111
Fax: (617) 918-1809
Toll free within Region 1: (888)
  372-7341

Region 2 (NJ, NY, PR, VI)
Environmental Protection Agency
290 Broadway
New York, NY 10007-1866
Phone: (212) 637-3000
Fax: (212) 637-3526

**Region 3 (DC, DE, MD, PA,
  VA, WV)**
Environmental Protection Agency
1650 Arch Street
Philadelphia, PA 19103-2029
Phone: (215) 814-5000
Fax: (215) 814-5103
Toll free: (800) 438-2474

**Region 4 (AL, FL, GA, KY, MS, NC,
  SC, TN)**
Environmental Protection Agency
Sam Nunn Atlanta Federal Center
61 Forsyth Street SW
Atlanta, GA 30303-3104
Phone: (404) 562-9900
Fax: (404) 562-8174
Toll free: (800) 241-1754

Region 5 (IL, IN, MI, MN, OH, WI)
Environmental Protection Agency
77 West Jackson Boulevard
Chicago, IL 60604-3507
Phone: (312) 353-2000
Fax: (312) 353-4135
Toll free within Region 5: (800)
  621-8431

Region 6 (AR, LA, NM, OK, TX)
Environmental Protection Agency
Fountain Place 12th Floor, Suite 1200
1445 Ross Avenue
Dallas, TX 75202-2733
Phone: (214) 665-2200
Toll free within Region 6: (800)
  887-6063

Region 7 (IA, KS, MO, NE)
Environmental Protection Agency
11201 Renner Blvd.
Lenexa, KS 66219
Phone: (913) 551-7003
Toll free: (800) 223-0425

Region 8 (CO, MT, ND, SD, UT, WY)
Environmental Protection Agency
1595 Wynkoop St.
Denver, CO 80202-1129
Phone: (303) 312-6312
Fax: (303) 312-6339
Toll free: (800) 227-8917
Email: r8eisc@epa.gov

Region 9 (AZ, CA, HI, NV)
Environmental Protection Agency
75 Hawthorne Street
San Francisco, CA 94105
Phone: (415) 947-8000
Fax: (415) 947-3553
Toll free in Region 9: (866) EPA-WEST
Email: r9.info@epa.gov

Region 10 (AK, ID, OR, WA)
Environmental Protection Agency
1200 Sixth Avenue, Suite 900
Seattle, WA 98101
Phone: (206) 553-1200
Fax: (206) 553-2955
Toll free: (800) 424-4372

Books

Carson, R. *Silent Spring (1962)*. Houghton Mifflin, Cambridge.

Colburn, T., Dumanoski, D., & Myers, J. P. (1996). *Our Stolen Future: Are We Threatening Our Fertility, Intelligence, and Survival? A Scientific Detective Story*; Dutton, New York.

Grandjean, P. (2015). *Only One Chance: How Environmental Pollution Impairs Brain Development and How to Protect the Brains of the Next Generation* (Environmental Ethics and Science Policy Series). Oxford University Press, Oxford.

Jackson, R., & Sinclair, S. (2012). *Designing Healthy Communities*. John Wiley and Sons, New York.

Landrigan, P., & Etzel, R., Eds. (2013). *Textbook of Children's Environmental Health*. Oxford University Press, Oxford.

Child Environmental Health Advocacy Groups

Children's Environmental Health Network   www.cehn.org
Healthy Child Healthy World   www.healthychild.org
Children's Environmental Health Network   www.cehn.org

Asthma and Air Pollution

Selected Journal Articles

Delamater, P. L., Finley, A. O., & Banerjee, S. (2012). An analysis of asthma hospitalizations, air pollution, and weather conditions in Los Angeles County, California. *Science of the Total Environment 425*, 110–118. doi: 10.1016/j.scitotenv.2012.02.015

Friedman, M. S., Powell, K. E., Hutwagner, L., Graham, L. M., & Teague, W. G. (2001). Impact of changes in transportation and commuting behaviors during the 1996 Summer Olympic Games in Atlanta on air quality and childhood asthma. *JAMA 285*(7), 897–905. PMID: 11180733.

Gauderman, W. J., Urman, R., Avol, E., Berhane, K., McConnell, R., Rappaport, E., Chang, R., Lurmann, F., & Gilliland, F. (2015). Association of improved air quality with lung development in children. *N Engl J Med 372*, 905–913. doi: 10.1056/NEJMoa1414123

Khreis, H., Kelly, C., Tate, J., Parslow, R., Lucas, K., & Nieuwenhuijsen, M. (2017). Exposure to traffic-related air pollution and risk of development of childhood asthma: A systematic review and meta-analysis. *Environ Int. 100*, 1–31. doi: 10.1016/j.envint.2016.11.012

Korten, I., Ramsey, K., & Latzin, P. (2017). Air pollution during pregnancy and lung development in the child. *Paediatr Respir Rev. 21*, 38–46. doi: 10.1016/j.prrv.2016.08.008.

Li, Y., Wang, W., Wang, J., Zhang, X., Lin, W., & Yang, Y. (2011). Impact of air pollution control measures and weather conditions on asthma during the 2008 Summer Olympic Games in Beijing. *Int J Biometeorol 55*(4), 547–554. doi: 10.1007/s00484-010-0373-6

Logan, W. P. (1953). Mortality in the London fog incident, 1952. *Lancet 1*, 336–338. PMID:13012086.

Pope, D. P., Mishra, V., Thompson, L., Siddiqui, A. R., Rehfuess, E. A., Weber. M., & Bruce, N. G. (2010). Risk of low birth weight and stillbirth associated with indoor air pollution from solid fuel use in developing countries. *Epidemiol Rev 32*, 70–81. doi: 10.1093/epirev/mxq005

Sly, P., & Flack, F. (2008). Susceptibility of children to environmental pollutants. *Annals NY Acad Sci 1140*, 163–183. doi: 10.1196/annals.1454.017

Wichmann, F. A., Müller, A., Busi, L. E., Cianni, N., Massolo, L., Schlink, U., Porta, A., & Sly, P. D.(2009). Increased asthma and respiratory symptoms in children exposed to petrochemical pollution. *J Allergy Clin Immunol 123*, 632–638. doi: 10.1016/j.jaci.2008.09.052.

Websites
Asthma and Outdoor Air Pollution,
    EPA-452-F-04-003   www3.epa.gov
AirNow   www.airnow.gov
Scorecard: The Pollution Information Site   www.scorecard.org

Childhood Cancer
Reviews
America's Children and the Environment, 2015   www.epa.gov

Selected Journal Articles

Chen, M., Chang, C. H., Tao, L., & Lu, C. (2015). Residential exposure to pesticides during childhood and childhood cancers: A meta-analysis. *Pediatrics 136*(4), 719–729. doi: 10.1542/peds.2015-0006.

Cohn, B. A., La Merrill, M., Krigbaum, N. Y., Yeh, G., Park, J. S., Zimmermann, L., & Cirillo, P. M. (2015). DDT exposure in utero and breast cancer. *J Clin Endocrinol Metab 100*(8), 2865–2867. doi: 10.1210/jc.2015-1841

Cohn, B. A., Wolff, M. S., Cirillo, P. M., & Sholtz, R. I. (2007). DDT and breast cancer in young women: new data on the significance of age at exposure. *Environmental Health Perspectives 115*(10), 1406–1414. PMID:17938728

Feychting, M., Plato, N., Nise, G., Ahlbom, A. (2001). Paternal occupational exposures and childhood cancer. *Environmental Health Perspectives 115*(12), 1787–1789.

IARC Monographs on the Evaluation of Carcinogenic Risks to Humans.
Geneva: World Health Organization, 2012. Retrieved from http://
monographs.iarc.fr/ENG/Classification/

Infante-Rivard, C., & Weichenthal, S. (2007). Pesticides and childhood
cancer: An update of Zahm and Ward's 1998 review. *J. Toxicol and
Environ Health Part B: Critical Reviews 10*(1–2), 81–99. PMID: 18074305

Landrigan, P. J., Schechter, C. B., Lipton, J. M., Fahs, M. C., &
Schwartz, J. (2002). Environmental pollutants and disease in
American children: Estimates of morbidity, mortality and costs
for lead poisoning, asthma, cancer and developmental diabetes.
Environmental Health Perspectives, 110, 721–728. PMID:12117650.

Pesatori, A. C., Consonni, D., Rubagotti, M., Grillo, P., & Bertazzi, P. A.
(2009). Cancer incidence in the population exposed to dioxin after
the "Seveso accident": Twenty years of follow-up. *Environ Health 8,*
39–47. doi: 10.1186/1476-069X-8-39. PMID: 19754930

Raaschou-Nielsen, O., Andersen, C. E., Andersen, H. P., Gravesen,
P., Lind, M., Schüz, J., & Ulbak, K. (2008). Domestic radon and
childhood cancer in Denmark. *Epidemiology, 19*(4), 536–543.
doi: 10.1097/EDE.0b013e318176bfcd. PMID: 18552587.

Warner, M., Mocarelli, P., Samuels, S., Needham, L., Brambilla, P., &
Eskenazi, B. (2011). Dioxin exposure and cancer risk in the Seveso
women's health study. *Environmental Health Perspectives, 119,* 1700–
1705. doi: 10.1289/ehp.1103720.

Endocrine Disruptors and Reproductive Disorders
Early Warnings

Carson, R. *(1962). Silent Spring.* Houghton Mifflin, Cambridge.

Colburn, T., Dumanoski, D., & Myers, J. P. (1996). *Our Stolen Future: Are
We Threatening Our Fertility, Intelligence, and Survival? A Scientific
Detective Story.* Dutton, New York.

Websites

European Commission, Endocrine Disruptors	www.ec.europa.eu
Environmental Working Group	www.ewg.org
National Institute of Environmental Health Sciences	www.niehs.nih.org
World Health Organization	www.who.int

Selected Documents and Journal Articles

Endocrine Society Scientific Statement 2009	www.endocrine.org
Pesticides and Endocrine Disruption	www.beyondpesticides.org

Barker, D. J. (2004). The developmental origins of adult disease. *J Am
Coll Nutr 23,* 588S–595S. PMID: 15640511.

Bergman, Å., Heindel, J. J., Kasten, T., Kidd, K. A., Jobling, S., Neira,
    M., Zoeller, R. T., Becher, G., Bjerregaard, P., Bornman, R., Brandt I,
    Kortenkamp,A., Muir, D., Drisse, M. N., Ochieng, R., Skakkebaek,
    N. E., Byléhn, A. S., Iguchi, T., Toppari, J., & Woodruff, T. J. (2013).
    The Impact of Endocrine Disruption: A Consensus Statement
    on the State of the Science. *Environ Health Perspect 121*, a104–6.
    doi: 10.1289/ehp.1205448.

Braun, J. M., Yolton, K., Dietrich, K. N., Hornung, R., Ye, X., Calafat,
    A. M., & Lanphear, B. P. (2009). Prenatal bisphenol A exposure and
    early childhood behavior. *Environmental Health Perspectives 117*,
    1945–1952. doi: 10.1289/ehp.0900979.

Burns, J. S., Williams, P. L., Sergeyev, O., Korrick, S. A., Lee, M. M.,
    Revich, B., Altshul, L., Del Prato, J. T., Humblet, O., Patterson, D. G.,
    Turner, W. E., Starovoytov, M., & Hauser, R. (2011). Serum dioxins
    and polychlorinated biphenyls are associated with growth among
    Russian boys. *Pediatrics 127*, e59–e68. doi: 10.1289/ehp.1103743.

Calafat, A. M., Ye, X., Wong, L. Y., Reidy, J. A., & Needham, L. L. (2008).
    Exposure of the U. S. population to bisphenol A and 4-tertiary-
    octylphenol: 2003–2004. *Environmental Health Perspectives 116*, 39–44.
    doi: 10.1289/ehp.10753.

Colborn, T., vom Saal, F. S., & Soto, A. M. (1993). Developmental
    effects of endocrine-disrupting chemicals in wildlife and
    humans. *Environmental Health Perspectives 101*, 378–384.
    PMCID: PMC1519860.

Engels S.M, Miodovnik, A., Canfield, R. L., Zhu, C., Silva, M. J.,
    Calafat, A. M., & Wolff, M. S. (2010). Prenatal phthalate exposure
    is associated with childhood behavior and executive functioning.
    Environ Health Perspect 118(4), 565–571. doi: 10.1289/ehp.0901470

Eisenberg, M. L., Hsieh, M. H., Walters, R. C., Krasnow, R., &
    Lipshultz, L. I. (2011). The relationship between anogenital
    distance, fatherhood, and fertility in adult men. *PLoS One 6*, e18973.
    doi: 10.1371/journal.pone.0018973.

Herbst, A. L., Ulfelder, H., & Poskanzer, D. C. (1971). Adenocarcinoma
    of the vagina: Association of maternal stilbestrol therapy with
    tumor appearance in young women. *N Engl J Med 284*, 878–881.

Herbstman, J. B., Sjödin, A., Kurzon, M., Lederman, S. A., Jones,
    R. S., Rauh, V., Needham, L. L., Tang, D., Niedzwiecki, M.,
    Wang, R. Y., & Perera, F. (2010). Prenatal exposure to PBDEs and
    neurodevelopment. *Environmental Health Perspectives 118*, 712–719.
    doi: 10.1289/ehp.0901340.

Hoffman, K., Webster, T. F., Sjödin, A., & Stapleton, H. M. (2010). Exposure to polyfluoroalkyl chemicals and attention deficit/hyperactivity disorder in U.S. children 12-15 years of age. *Environmental Health Perspectives 118*, 1762–1767. doi: 10.1038/jes.2016.11.

Masuo, Y., & Ishido, M. (2011). Neurotoxicity of endocrine disruptors: Possible involvement in brain development and neurodegeneration. *J Toxicol Environ Health B 14*, 346–369. doi: 10.1080/10937404.2011.578557.

Mendiola, J., Stahlhut, R. W., Jørgensen, N., Liu, F., & Swan, S. H. (2011). Shorter anogenital distance predicts poorer semen quality in young men in Rochester, New York. *Environmental Health Perspectives 119*, 958–963. doi: 10.1289/ehp.1103421.

Singh, S., Li, S. S. (2012). Epigenetic effects of environmental chemicals bisphenol A and phthalates. *Int J Mol Sci 13*, 10143–10153. doi: 10.3390/ijms130810143.

Swan, S. H. (2000). Intrauterine exposure to diethylstilbestrol: Long-term effects in humans. *APMIS 108*, 793–804.

Swan, S. H., Liu, F., Hines, M., Kruse, R. L., Wang, C., Redmon, J. B., Sparks, A., Weiss, B. (2010). Prenatal phthalate exposure and reduced masculine play in boys. *Int J Androl 33*, 259–269. doi: 10.1111/j.1365-2605.2009.01019.x.

Swan, S. H., & Weiss, B. (2012). Phthalates: What they are and why they raise concerns about human health. In R. H. Friis (Ed.), *Praeger Handbook of Environmental Health* (pp. 453–473). Santa Barbara: ABC-CLIO.

Turyk, M. E., Persky, V. W., Imm, P., Knobeloch, L., Chatterton, R., & Anderson, H. A. (2008). Hormone disruption by PBDEs in adult male sport fish consumers. *Environmental Health Perspectives 116*, 1635–1641. doi: 10.1289/ehp.11707.

World Health Organization. (2010). *Dioxins and their effects on human health*. Fact sheet N° 225. Geneva: World Health Organization.

Childhood Obesity

Built Environment and Health
Impact of the Built Environment on Health,
Centers for Disease Control
and Prevention   www.cdc.gov/healthyplaces
Robert Woods Johnson Foundation   rwjf.org

Jackson, R., & Sinclair, S. (2012). *Designing Healthy Communities*. New Yok: John Wiley and Sons.

Selected Journal Articles

American Academy of Pediatrics Committee on Environmental Health. (2009). The built environment: Designing communities to promote physical activity in children. *Pediatrics 123*, 1591–1598. doi:10.1542/peds.2009-0750.

Behl, M., Rao, D., Aagaard-Tillery, K., Davidson, T. L., Levin, E. D., Slotkin, T. A., Srinivasan, S., Wallinga, D., White, M. F., Walker, V. R., Thayer, K. A., & Holloway, A. C. (2013). Evaluation of the association between maternal smoking, childhood obesity, and metabolic disorders: A National Toxicology Program Workshop Report. *Environmental Health Perspectives 121*, 170–180. doi: 10.1289/ehp.1205404.

Ino, T. (2010). Maternal smoking during pregnancy and offspring obesity: Meta-analysis. *Pediatr Int 52*, 94–99. doi: 10.1111/j.1442-200X.2009.02883.x.

La Merrill, M., & Birnbaum, L. S. (2011). Childhood obesity and environmental chemicals. *Mt Sinai J Med 78*, 22–48. PMID: 21259261

La Merrill M, Emond C, Kim MJ, Antignac JP, Le Bizec B, Clément K, Birnbaum LS, & Barouki R. (2013). Toxicological function of adipose tissue: Focus on persistent organic pollutants. *Environmental Health Perspectives 121*, 162–169. doi: 10.1289/ehp.1205485.

Oken, E., Levitan, E. B., & Gillman, M. W. (2008). Maternal smoking during pregnancy and child overweight: Systematic review and meta-analysis. *Int J Obes 32*, 201–210. doi: 10.1038/sj.ijo.0803760.

Rahman, T., Cushing, R. A., & Jackson, R. J. J. (2011). Contribution of built environment to childhood obesity. *Mt Sinai J Med 78*, 49–57. doi: 10.1002/msj.20235.

Somm, E., Schwitzgebel, V. M., Vauthay, D. M., Camm, E. J., Chen, C. Y., Giacobino, J. P., Sizonenko, S. V., Aubert, M. L., & Hüppi, P. S. (2008). Prenatal nicotine exposure alters early pancreatic islet and adipose tissue development with consequences on the control of body weight and glucose metabolism later in life. *Endocrinology 149*, 6289–6299. doi: 10.1210/en.2008-0361.

Thayer, K. A., Heindel, J. J., Bucher, J. R., & Gallo, M. A. (2012). Role of environmental chemicals in diabetes and obesity: A National Toxicology Program Workshop Report. *Environmental Health Perspectives 120*, 779–789. doi: 10.1289/ehp.1104597.

Trasande, L., Attina, T. M., & Blustein, J. (2012). Association between urinary bisphenol A concentration and obesity prevalence in children and adolescents. *JAMA 308*, 1113–1121. PMID: 22990270

Environmental Toxins and Brain Development

Book

Grandjean, P. (2015). *Only One Chance: How Environmental Pollution Impairs Brain Development and How to Protect the Brains of the Next Generation* (Environmental Ethics and Science Policy Series). Oxford University Press, London.

Selected Journal Articles

Bellinger, D. C. (2011). The protean toxicities of lead: New chapters in a familiar story. *Int J Environ Res Public Health 8*, 2593–2628. doi: 10.3390/ijerph8072593.

Blumberg, S. J., Bramlett, M. D., Kogan, M. D., Schieve, L. A., Jones, J. R., Lu, M. C. (2013). Changes in prevalence of parent-reported autism spectrum disorder in school-aged U.S. children: 2007 to 2011–2012. *National Health Statistics Reports, 6.* PMID: 24988818.

Braun, J. M., Kahn, R. S., Froehlich, T., Auinger, P., & Lanphear, B. P. (2006). Exposures to environmental toxicants and attention deficit hyperactivity disorder in U.S. children. *Environmental Health Perspectives 114*, 1904–1909. doi: 10.1289/ehp.9478

Brown, J. S. (2009). Effects of bisphenol-A and other endocrine disruptors compared with abnormalities of schizophrenia: An endocrine-disruption theory of schizophrenia. *Schizophrenia Bull 35*, 256–278. PMID: 18245062.

Ciesielski, T., Weuve, J., Bellinger, D. C., Schwartz, J., Lanphear, B., & Wright, R. O. (2012). Cadmium exposure and neurodevelopmental outcomes in U.S. children. *Environmental Health Perspectives 120*, 758–763. doi: 10.1289/ehp.1104152.

Grandjean, P., & Landrigan, P. J. (2006). Developmental neurotoxicity of industrial chemicals. *Lancet 368*, 2167–2178. PMID: 17174709.

Grandjean, P., & Landrigan, P. J. (2014). Neurobehavioural effects of developmental toxicity. *Lancet Neurol 13*, 330–338. doi: 10.1016/S1474-4422(13)70278-3.

Kim, B-N., Cho, S-C., Kim, Y., Shin, M. S., Yoo, H. J., Kim, J. W., Yang, Y. H., Kim, H. W., Bhang, S. Y., & Hong, Y. C. (2009). Phthalate exposure and attention deficit/hyperactivity disorder in school-age children. *Biol Psychiat 66*, 958–963. doi: 10.1016/j.biopsych.2009.07.034.

Landrigan, P. J. (2010). What causes autism? Exploring the environmental contribution. *Curr Opin Pediatr 22*, 219–225. doi: 10.1097/MOP.0b013e328336eb9a.

Lee, D-H., Jacobs, D. R., & Porta, M. (2007). Association of serum concentrations of persistent organic pollutants with the prevalence of learning disability and attention deficit disorder. *J Epidemiol Comm Health 61*, 591–596. PMID: 17568050

Rauh, V., Garfinkel, R., Perera, F. P., Andrews, H. F., Hoepner, L., Barr, D. B., Whitehead, R., Tang, D., & Whyatt, R. W. (2006). Impact of prenatal chlorpyrifos exposure on neurodevelopment in the first 3 years of life among inner-city children. *Pediatrics 118*, e1845–5. PMID: 17116700.

Underwood, E. (2017). The polluted brain. *Science 355*(6523), 342–245. doi: 10.1126/science.355.6323.342.

Volk, H. E., Lurmann, F., Penfold, B., Hertz-Picciotto, I., McConnell, R., & Campbell, D. B. (2013). Traffic-related air pollution, particulate matter, and autism. *JAMA Psychiatry 70*, 71–77. doi: 10.1001/jamapsychiatry.2013.266.

Windham, G. C., Zhang, L., Gunier, R., Croen, L. A., & Grether, J. K. (2006). Autism spectrum disorders in relation to distribution of hazardous air pollutants in the San Francisco Bay area. *Environmental Health Perspectives 114*, 1438–1444. PMID: 16966102.

Epigenetics and New Technologies—Biomarkers of Disease and Exposure

Selected Journal Articles

Andra, S. S., Austin, C., & Arora, M. (2016). The tooth exposome in children's health research. *Current Opinions Pediatr 28*(2), 221–227. doi: 10.1097/MOP.0000000000000327.

Arora, M., Hare, D., Austin, C., Smith, D. R., Doble, P. (2011). Spatial distribution of manganese in enamel and coronal dentine of human primary teeth. *Sci Total Environ 409*(7), 1315–1319. doi: 10.1016/j.scitotenv.2010.12.018.

Carter, C. J., & Blizard, R. A. (2016). Autism genes are selectively targeted by environmental pollutants including pesticides, heavy metals, bisphenol A, phthalates and many others in food, cosmetics, or household products. *Neurochem Int*, pii: S0197-0186(16)30197-8. doi: 10.1016/j.neuint.2016.10.011.

Knopick, V. S., Maccani, M. A., Francazio, S., & McGeary, J. E. 2012). The epigenetics of maternal cigarette smoking during pregnancy and effects on child development. *Development and Psychopathology 24*(4), 1377–1390. doi: 10.1017/S0954579412000776.

Latham, K. E., Sapienza, C., Engel, N. (2012). The epigenetic Lorax: Gene–environment interactions in human health. *Epigenenomics 4*(4), 383–402. doi: 10.2217/epi.12.31.

Modabbernia, A., A, Velthorst, E., Gennings, C., De Haan, L., Austin, C., Sutterland, A., Mollon, J., Frangou, S., Wright, R., Arora, M., & Reichenberg, A. (2016). Early life metal exposure and schizophrenia: A proof of concept study using novel tooth-matrix biomarkers. *Eur Psychiatry 36*, 1–8. doi: 10.1016/j.eurpsy.2016.03.006.

Morishita, H., & Arora, M. (2017). Tooth-matrix biomarkers to reconstruct critical periods of brain plasticity. *Trends Neurosci 40*(1), 1–3. doi: 10.1016/j.tins.2016.11.003.

Power, C., & Jefferis, B. J. (2002). Fetal environment and subsequent obesity: A study of maternal smoking. *Int J Epidemiol 31*(2), 413–419. PMID: 11980805.

Rauh, V. A., Perera, F. P., Horton, M. K., Whyatt, R. M., Bansal, R., Hao, X., Liu, J., Barr, D. B., Slotkin, T. A., & Peterson, B. S. (2012). Brain anomalies in children exposed prenatally to a common organophosphate pesticide. *Proc Natl Acad Sci USA. 109*, 7871–7876. doi: 10.1073/pnas.1203396109.

Legislation

European Commission, REACH	www.ec.europa.eu
The Frank R. Lautenberg Chemical Safety for the 21st Century Act	www.epa.gov
Clean Water Act of 1972	www.epa.gov
Clean Air Act of 1970/1977/1990	www.epa.gov
Safe Drinking Water Act	www.epa.gov

Selected Journal Article

Landrigan, P. J., & Goldman, L. R. (2011). Children's vulnerability to toxic chemicals: A challenge and opportunity to strengthen health and environmental policy. *Health Aff 30*, 842–850. doi: 10.1377/hlthaff.2011.0151.

Organic Gardening

Bradley, F. M., Ellis, B. W., & Martin, D. L.(2009) *The Organic Gardener's Handbook of Natural Pest and Disease Control: A Complete Guide to Maintaining a Healthy Garden and Yard the Earth-Friendly Way.* Emmaus PA: Rodale Press.

Bradley, F. M., Phillips E., & Ellis, B. (2009). *Rodale's Ultimate Encyclopedia of Organic Gardening: The Indispensable Green Resource for Every Gardener.* Emmaus PA: Rodale Press.

Martin, D. (2014). *Basic Organic Gardening: A Beginner's Guide to Starting a Health Garden.* Emmaus PA: Rodale Press.

Pesticides

Resource Groups

Beyond Pesticides	www.beyondpesticides.org
Environmental Working Group	www.ewg.org
Medline Plus	www.medlineplus.gov
National Institutes of Environmental Health	www.nih.niehs.gov
National Pesticide Information Center	www.npic.orst.edu
Toxnet	www.toxnet.nlm.nih.gov

Selected Reviews and Journal Articles

American Academy of Pediatrics Council on Environmental Health. (2012). Pesticides. In R. A. Etzel & S. J. Balk (Eds.), *Pediatric Environmental Health* (3rd ed.). Elk Grove Village, IL: American Academy of Pediatrics. ISBN-13: 978-1-58110-653-4

Bouchard, M. F., Chevrier, J., Harley, K. G., Kogut, K., Vedar, M., Calderon, N., Trujillo, C., Johnson, C., Bradman A, Barr, D. B., & Eskenazi, B. (2011). Prenatal exposure to organophosphate pesticides and IQ in 7-year-old children. *Environmental Health Perspectives 119*, 1189–1195. doi: 10.1289/ehp.1003185.

Centers for Disease Control and Prevention. (2009). *Fourth Report on Human Exposure to Environmental Chemicals.* Atlanta, GA: US Department of Health and Human Services, Centers for Disease Control and Prevention. Retrieved from http://www.cdc.gov/exposurereport/

Cohn, B. A., La Merrill, M., Krigbaum, N. Y., Yeh, G., Park, J. S., Zimmermann, L., & Cirillo, P. M. (2015). DDT exposure in utero and breast cancer. *J Clin Endocrinol Metab 100*(8), 2865–2867. doi: 10.1210/jc.2015-1841

Cohn, B. A., Wolff, M. S., Cirillo, P. M., & Sholtz, R. I. (2007). DDT and breast cancer in young women: new data on the significance of age at exposure. *Environmental Health Perspectives 115*(10), 1406–1414. PMID:17938728

Engel, S. M., Wetmur, J., Chen, J., Zhu, C., Barr, D. B., Canfield, R. L., & Wolff, M. S. (2011). Prenatal exposure to organophosphates, paraoxonase 1, and cognitive development in childhood.

Environmental Health Perspectives 119, 1182–1188. doi: 10.1289/
ehp.1003183.

Grandjean, P., Harari, R., Barr, D. B., & Debes, F. (2006). Pesticide
exposure and stunting as independent predictors of
neurobehavioral deficits in Ecuadorian school children. *Pediatrics
117*, e546–e556. PMID: 16510633

Karr, C., Solomon, G. M., & Brock-Utne, A. (2007). Health effects of
common home, lawn and garden pesticides. *Pediatr Clin North Am
54*, 63–80. doi: 10.1016/j.pcl.2006.11.005

Lu, C., Toepel, K., Irish, R., Fenske, R. A., Barr, D. B., & Bravo, R. (2006).
Organic diets significantly lower children's dietary exposure to
organophosphorus pesticides. *Environmental Health Perspectives 114*,
260–263. PMID: 16451864.

Rauh, V. A., Arunajadai, S., Horton, M., Perera, F., Hoepner, L., Barr,
D. B., & Whyatt, R. (2011). Seven-year neurodevelopmental scores
and prenatal exposure to chlorpyrifos, a common agricultural
pesticide. *Environmental Health Perspectives 119*, 1196–1201.
doi: 10.1289/ehp.1003160.

Rauh, V. A., Perera, F. P., Horton, M. K., Whyatt, R. M., Bansal, R.,
Hao, X., Liu, J., Barr, D. B., Slotkin, T. A., & Peterson, B. S. (2012).
Brain anomalies in children exposed prenatally to a common
organophosphate pesticide. *Proc Natl Acad Sci USA 109*, 7871–7876.
doi: 10.1073/pnas.1203396109.

Roberts, J. R., & Karr, C. J. (2012). American Academy of Pediatrics
Council on Environmental Health. Pesticide exposure in children.
Technical Report. *Pediatrics 130*, e1765–e1788. doi: 10.1542/
peds.2012-2758.

U.S. Department of Housing and Urban Development. (2006). *Healthy
Homes Issues: Pesticides in the Home—Use, Hazards, and Integrated Pest
Management*. Retrieved from http://portal.hud.gov/hudportal/
documents/huddoc?id=DOC_12484.pdf

News Articles

Hakim, D. (2016, October 29). Uncertain Harvest: Doubts about the
promised bounty of genetically modified crops. *The New York Times.*

Hakim, D. (2016, December 16). Uncertain Harvest: This pesticide
is prohibited in Britain. Why is it still being exported? *The
New York Times.*

Hakim, D. (2016, December 31). Uncertain Harvest: Scientists loved and
loathed by an agrochemical giant. *The New York Times.*

Tobacco

Reports

Centers for Disease Control and Prevention. (2010). *How Tobacco Smoke Causes Disease: The Biology and Behavioral Basis for Smoking-Attributable Disease: A Report of the Surgeon General.* Atlanta, GA: National Center for Chronic Disease Prevention and Health Promotion; Office on Smoking and Health.

Centers for Disease Control and Prevention. (2016). *E-Cigarette Use Among Youth and Young Adults: A Report of the Surgeon General.* Atlanta, GA: National Center for Chronic Disease Prevention and Health Promotion; Office on Smoking and Health.

Recent Reviews

Carter, B. D., Abnet, C. C., Feskanich, D., Freedman, N. D., Hartge, P., Lewis, C. E., Ockene, J. K., Prentice, R. L., Speizer, F. E., Thun, M. J., & Jacobs, E. J. (2015). Smoking and mortality—Beyond established causes. New Engl J Med, *372,* 631–640. doi: 10.1056/NEJMsa1407211.

Monti, D, Kuzemchak, M. & Politi, M. *The Effects of Smoking on Health Insurance Decisions Under the Affordable Care Act.* Center for Health Economics and Policy, Institute for Public Health at Washington University. Available at: https://publichealth.wustl.edu/wp-content/uploads/2016/04/The-Effects-of-Smoking-on-Health-Insurance-Decisions-Under-the-Affordable-Care-Act_updated.pdf. [Accessed 2 August 2017].

Websites and Fact Sheets

CDC Fact Sheets: Health Effects of
Cigarette Smoking and others   www.cdc.gov
Multiple fact sheets on tobacco and health   betobaccofree.hhs.gov
Electronic cigarettes: An Overview
of Key Issues   tobaccofreek

INDEX